WINDOWS ON THE MIND

WINDOWS ON THE MIND

Reflections on the Physical Basis of Consciousness

ERICH HARTH

WILLIAM MORROW AND COMPANY, INC.

New York   1982

Library of Congress Cataloging in Publication Data

Harth, Erich.
  Windows on the mind.

  Includes bibliographical references and index.
  1. Consciousness.   2. Intellect.   3. Brain.
I. Title.
QP411.H37   153   81-11158
ISBN 0-688-00751-1   AACR2

Printed in the United States of America

First Edition

1 2 3 4 5 6 7 8 9 10

Grateful acknowledgment is made to the following individuals, publishers, and institutions for permission to reproduce visual material:

The University of Illinois, for permission to reproduce three figures from *The Isocortex of Man* by Percival Bailey and Gerhardt von Bonin, © 1951 by the University of Illinois Press. Board of Editors: A. C. Ivy, O. F. Kampmeier, Isaak Schour, and E. R. Serles.

The Williams & Wilkins Company, for permission to reproduce a figure from *Human Neuroanatomy* by Dr. Malcolm B. Carpenter, © 1964, the Williams & Wilkins Company, Baltimore.

Robert J. Collier and Academic Press, Inc., for permission to reproduce a figure from *Optical Holography* by Robert J. Collier, Christoph B. Burckhardt, and Lawrence H. Lin, © 1971 by Academic Press, Inc.

The Visual Artists and Galleries Association, Inc., for permission to reproduce "Flatworms" by M. C. Escher, © Beeldrecht, Amsterdam/VAGA, New York, Collection Haags Gemeentemuseum—The Hague, 1982.

Dr. Leon D. Harmon and Bell Laboratories, for permission to reproduce Dr. Harmon's computer-generated image of Lincoln.

David B. Brobecker, for permission to reproduce his photo of an anglerfish.

BOOK DESIGN BY MICHAEL MAUCERI

To *Dorothy, Peter, and Rick*

CONTENTS

3

HANG-UPS IN NEUROSCIENCE

Some traditional disputes are examined here. They are important in directing our attention to certain features of brain function and away from others.

4

A VIEW FROM BELOW

A closer look at the physical system with greater emphasis on the role of peripheral brain structures.

WINDOWS ON THE MIND

1

A SIMPLEMINDED VIEW FROM A DISTANCE

I had risen up to look into the jar, but now I was sunk in my chair, speechless. My eyes were fixed upon that jar as I tried to comprehend that these pieces of gunk bobbing up and down had caused a revolution, in physics and quite possibly changed the course of civilization. There it was.

—From Steven Levy's account of finding Einstein's brain.

He tells us that he had known three cubebs taken every day to have a wonderful effect in invigorating the memory . . .
Should this boon be reserved for the human race, it will be humane and pious to wish, that it may not be found out, until men shall cease to concentrate the utmost force of their faculties, in discovering new modes of public and private oppression, and new instruments for inflicting pain and death upon each other.

—BENJAMIN RUSH (1746–1813), Two Essays on the Mind

Introduction

If I had to state the subject matter of this book in one sentence, I would say it deals with the question "What kind of a thing is man?" By this I really mean to ask, "What makes me fundamentally different from an oxygen atom, a locomotive, or a gorilla?"

The three examples are not chosen frivolously. For it is from just these three classes of things that we must distinguish ourselves: the natural inanimate object, the machine, and our nearest relatives in the animal kingdom. In turn, they conjure up metaphors which some of us may find disturbing: man the microcosm, man the computer, man the ape.

Where do we look for our mark of distinction? There was a time when we believed our bodies were inhabited by spirits and humors. People had souls. Our hearts were capable of generating love, and we could hate with our guts. But science has taught us that a heart is just a pump and our guts a chemical factory. And so the spirits have been exorcized from one part of our bodies after another, "from whence," in the words of Warren McCulloch, the late MIT psychiatrist-cybernetician, "they went straight to our heads, like bats to the belfry."[1] Here they still reside in this untidy attic of science amid a clutter of some of the oldest notions about ourselves and some of the latest facts. And here we again attempt to uncover the essence of our own nature in the vast machinery of our brain or in the unique abilities and predilections we call our mind.

Brain and mind. Few would contend that one can be human without these, so we shall make them the focus of our study. Unfortunately, this does not narrow the field of our inquiry because in considering the mind, we bring in the full range of interactions between the individual and the rest of the universe. This leaves out very little, and the task appears hopeless. It would have to include an assessment of man's works, both noble and ignoble. Surely it is significant that no other creatures, no other systems, to use that dreary engineering term, are able to write a *Hamlet,* or a "Kreutzer Sonata," or conceive of concentration camps. Perhaps it is only by these creations that we can define the human animal. But we will try to look for attributes that are more primitive and more fundamental.

The human brain is approximately three pounds of living tissue consisting of blood vessels, some membranous linings, some fluid-filled cavities, and many billions of specialized cells, the most important of which are about ten billion neurons. These form a communications network of unmatched complexity.

Apart from its "housekeeping functions" of overseeing all the vital processes in our bodies, the brain is the unique organizer that imposes a *oneness** on the various parts of the body. It is the originator and the repository of *selfhood*. It alone can make the distinction between that which is part of *me* and the rest of the world. Curiously, it has no sensation of its own existence. I never see my own brain, it makes no noises like my stomach, I can't feel its functioning like the pulsebeat of my heart, I can't even squeeze it, pinch it, palpate it. It is the most hidden and the most unobtrusive part of my body. It never hurts; a surgeon's knife could slice through it without causing any discomfort. Yet it is fiercely protective of that which it defines as its own.

If we could define mind as easily, many books would never have been written, including this one. But we must not delude ourselves into thinking that the problem is one of finding a definition, of coining the right phrase that will clear up the puzzle. I need not define what I know only too well and what, by inference, you have no trouble understanding. My sensations of pleasure and pain, and the hopes and fears that go with them, are a piece of my mind. So are all my wondering and guessing; my inclination to explore, take risks, invent, make puns, dream; my feeling of selfhood, and the contemplation of all my feelings, and my analysis of my contemplation. Still, mind may not be a thing apart but merely an activity, a mode of operation of the physical brain. Language misleads us into thinking that every noun is a thing, and that things are endowed with permanence and a set of enduring aspects of their own. We are truly baffled when someone asks us what happens to a person's lap when he stands up. We must guard against this tendency of mistaking the aspect of an object for the object itself.

It is likewise a mistake to believe that it is always *matter* which lends an object its permanence and individuality. Molecules are continuously entering and leaving a living system. Dying cells are replaced by new ones, and the material making up a cell is spent and replaced. The substance that was *me* ten years ago has mostly departed from my body and can no longer be responsible for my selfhood. What has endured is form and function, not matter.

Is mind then an aspect, a function of the physical brain? This seems almost to be an inevitable conclusion, but it does not fully satisfy our intellect. Mind is like no other property of physical systems. It is not

* Throughout the text, words are italicized either for emphasis or to indicate that they are technical terms. Most of the latter are defined in a glossary at the end of the book.

just that we don't know the mechanisms that give rise to it. We have difficulty seeing how *any* mechanism can give rise to it. This, in short, is the problem Schopenhauer has called the *world knot*.

The structure of the brain and the physical processes we can observe in it are the subject matter of neuroanatomy and neurophysiology, respectively. These studies have been immensely fruitful in recent decades, but they have been slow in shedding light on the old question of the brain's relation to the human mind. We will discuss this at length later after having reviewed some fundamental facts about the brain. For now, I wish to give only a bit of the flavor of the controversy and some of the standard positions. The problem cannot even be stated without using words or phrases that offend one school of thought or another. According to one philosophy, the problem doesn't even exist.

The brain is generally viewed as a very complicated and delicate *machine* whose functioning we are trying to understand. We are still very far from such an understanding, but let us be bold and suppose that at some future time we will understand the brain as well as we now do the heart, or the lung, or the kidneys. We would then know how information filters in through our senses; how it is processed (whatever that means); how memories are stored and recovered, skills learned, and decisions made; and how our muscles, glands, and all vital functions are controlled. We may still not know how to account for such things as thoughts and the sensations we associate with consciousness.

This impasse led René Descartes (1596–1650) to postulate two separate existences, the *body* and the *mind*.[2] Between these two we may readily account for almost anything, and that is the strength of this approach, which is known as *dualism*. But it has its weaknesses. For the mind to serve any useful function it must be able to have an effect on the brain. If I want to sit down and write a letter, this *want* must cause the brain to send signals to the appropriate muscles. To a physicist this is a disconcerting thought because it would mean that a nonphysical entity, the mind, is able to exert a physical influence on the body.

The materialist school of philosophy holds that the concept of a mind existing apart from the brain must be rejected as metaphysical. The late Oxford philosopher, Gilbert Ryle,[3] called it derisively the "ghost in the machine" or the "horse in the locomotive." According to the materialist school, all phenomena such as sensations, emotions, volition will in time be identified with specific physical processes in the brain. This school is best characterized by the following statement by the neurophysiologist J. Z. Young:

> Consider that without leaving the topic of the brain we can at least begin to discuss many, perhaps all, human activities. The method I am going to suggest as a working basis is to organize *all* our talk about human powers and capacities around knowledge of what the brain does. When the philosopher studies the way in which people think, let him consider what activity this represents in the brain: for certainly there is some. When the theologian studies the fact that human beings tend to organize their activities around statements about gods, let him consider the activity that this involves in the brain . . .[4]

This position has a certain neatness and compactness, but again we are left dissatisfied. I fail to find in it an explanation for *my* sensations of joy or fear. Young is purposely vague when he talks of "human activities," and I am left to wonder if any machine, however complex, can worry about its safety or enjoy being oiled.

Problems of this sort are generally avoided by keeping apart questions about *mind,* on the one hand, and about *body*, on the other. We do the same with science and religion, overlooking the fact that the two disciplines make statements about the same universe. Similarly, we observe here two routes over the same territory, but very little common ground.

Neurophysiology and neuroanatomy have been the main avenues of approach to knowledge about the physical brain. More recently, other sciences, including physics and mathematics, have joined a broader front of disciplines going under the name of *neuroscience.* When questions of sensation or consciousness are touched on at all—which does not happen very often—scientists generally resort to a traditional *reductionist* argument like the materialist view given above or they adopt some form of dualist approach.

Meanwhile, those thinking and writing about the mind have been just as unconcerned about the brain. It is only natural for someone who is interested in problems of human behavior to look for relationships between patterns of action and such psychological elements as wants, drives, and emotions rather than attempt, as Young has suggested, to delve into the hopelessly complex maze of brain circuits.

This schism between our approaches to the physical and what we can call the psychological self has some deplorable aspects. The majority of neuroscientists are naturally drawn to the primitive, machine-like aspects of the brain, leaving it to others to *philosophize* about such things as sensations, emotions, and consciousness. This unconcern with the "higher functions" may be responsible for the insensitivity scientists sometimes exhibit toward the pain inflicted on laboratory animals.

On the other hand, preoccupation with the psychological self has spawned some doctrines, practices, and cults which fly in the face of scientific knowledge that has been painstakingly gathered over centuries. Some of these doctrines originated at the outer fringes of science or beyond, but lately have come to dominate popular thinking and have even made inroads into the scientific community.

The dividing line between science and pseudoscience, between knowledge and superstition, is not always well defined. Different people would place the boundary at different locations. A field called *parapsychology* must be mentioned here because it is sometimes considered a legitimate scientific study of "mental phenomena," and because its findings, if true, would invalidate many of our concepts concerning the interdependence of mind and matter.

Among the phenomena claimed by parapsychologists are extrasensory perception (ESP), or the gathering of information without the aid of senses; telekinesis, or motion caused without the help of physical agency; and clairvoyance, or the ability to obtain knowledge in seeming defiance of time and space.

Two features characterize this field and distinguish it from traditional scientific approaches. There is among parapsychologists a general unconcern with the physical basis of the phenomena they report. Secondly, very little attempt is made to formulate laws and to seek regularities that might serve as a basis for understanding. The phenomena themselves are usually of a nature that makes duplication and verification by other investigators difficult if not impossible.

Our uncertainty regarding the nature of mind has always provided the incentive for numerous superstitions and cults. We have today a greater profusion of these than at any other time in the past. Books abound with tales of the occult and accounts of mental practices that are of dubious value. We live in an era in which our lives are wholly dependent on a great variety of advanced technologies, but public regard for scientific thought is probably at a low ebb.

I should explain at this point what I mean by *science*. The word conjures up a host of reactions, some favorable but many negative. In the minds of many, science has come to mean devices for mass destruction and the precarious balance of terror. The image of science I would like to convey instead is that of a well-tended garden, not an arsenal of technological marvels. The scientist is more a laborer than a magician. His task is the careful cultivation and gathering of knowledge gained through the observation of the world around him and of himself. Science is the continual sifting and reexamining of that knowledge. It is the organization and extension of knowledge through the application of rational mental processes, and it leads to the intellectual experience we call understanding. This, more than anything else, distinguishes science from all other pursuits.

To approach our task scientifically thus means only that we will look and examine and—where possible—try to understand. We will look upon the human mind not as a source of parlor tricks and powers to wield over other people or even over ourselves, but rather we will search for the qualities of the human mind in the uniqueness of man's physical nature. The search must begin at the crossroads of mind and body, the human brain.

Of myths and matter

The brain presents two seemingly irreconcilable aspects: It is a material body, exhibiting all the physical properties of matter, and it possesses a set of faculties and attributes, collectively called mind, that are not found in any other physical system.

The conceptual gap between these two aspects has not always been as profound as it seems today. In the animistic view of nature held in primitive societies, spirits resided in all matter and were responsible for most events observed in man's physical surroundings. Gradually man became more aware of certain immutable regularities that govern material objects. The study of these *laws* grew into physical science, and caprice and volition were expurgated from matter.

In this section I want to sketch very briefly how our views of the material universe have been fashioned. Ultimately the physical laws will have to be made accountable for the actions of the physical brain, and these in turn will have to be matched to the many aspects of human nature. We are still far from having accomplished any of these goals.

The exploration of physical surroundings is an activity we observe in all higher forms of life. We may therefore safely conclude that man from the very beginning has dedicated his wits to learning more about the world around him. His success in this venture has been enormous, while to this day the nature of his own observing self has remained largely unexplored.

The most primitive knowledge derived from the observation of nature is the fact of its constancy. The scenery I observe this second will still be here when I blink my eyes and look again. The mountains, the valley, the river whose images faded with the coming of night will be here at sunrise. This predictability and lack of sensory caprice was probably taken by primitive man as evidence that outside his body there existed a *world* independent of his own existence but in part reachable by his senses.

A second fact, complementary to and almost contradicting the first, emerges immediately: The world is a world of change. The mountain is not a dead slag heap but is covered with trees and shrubs that grow leaves, drop leaves, grow flowers, bear fruit, and die.

The task of every living thing in this world is to become attuned to these changes and turn them to its advantage. The animal knows where to find food, how to elude its predator, how to migrate with the changing seasons. Such knowledge may be instinctual or may be the result of learning.

In this duality of permanence and change, the permanent has often been identified with matter, while change retained a certain mysterious quality, something that had to be explained. One Greek school of philosophy, that of the Eleatics, suggested that change was beyond comprehension and hence was illusory. Only the permanent had reality.

Man's ambitions have made his interactions with the environment more far-ranging and more daring than those of any animal. To succeed he had to become the most painstaking observer of nature. To observe the world of change is to be prepared for change. With increased knowledge the range of man's activities also widened, and his need for knowledge increased further. The Bible story of his expulsion from the Garden of Eden after tasting fruit from the tree of knowledge can be understood as an early realization that the acquisition of knowledge cannot be reversed. Our intelligence, the size of our brain, have become our ecological niche, as body size had been that of the dinosaurs. It may be that—just as *they* had to follow their evolutionary cul-de-sac all the way to extinction—our dependence on the brain will lead us to a similar end. On the other hand, we may hope that, unlike sheer size or heavy armor, our brain may yet *think* its way out of the dilemmas and problems it has created for mankind: the threats of overpopulation and mass destruction. At any rate, it is my belief that there is no alternative to using our intelligence to the fullest, while hoping that benevolence and a sense of self-preservation will prevail. Our reasoning may lead us at times to forgo temporarily some knowledge in a limited area if we foresee a high risk of detrimental consequences. In the long run, however, I doubt that ignorance can ever again become our salvation.

The history of our acquisition of knowledge has not followed a straight course. The first steps were faltering, and man's curiosity often led to bewilderment. Beyond fashioning tools, controlling fire, and learning the rhythm of seasonal changes, there were just too many things to confound his mind. Besides the regularities that he learned to recognize and turn to his advantage, much in nature happened unpredictably, often disastrously. There was something in this caprice which reminded him of human actions. We can surmise that this perhaps led primitive man to attribute such phenomena to *spirits,* who for reasons of their own could *will* floods, droughts, and plagues.

In this *animistic* world picture, the worlds of physical phenomena and of spirits were one. Spirits resided in the objects they were controlling, or close by, and the gods—like those of ancient Greece—had form and substance and were vulnerable even though immortal.

But man never put his fate entirely into the hands of the spirits. He learned to make metals and observed the stars carefully to anticipate the coming of the seasons. He discovered the lodestone and invented gunpowder. At the same time, he kept perfecting his language and, with the invention of writing, managed to extend over space and time his ability to communicate with his fellows.

Conjecturing a little further in this sketch of the maturing of man's conception of nature, we can imagine that his curiosity about events then shifted to the spirits controlling them. Why did He send this drought? How can we induce Him (or Her—deities came in both sexes) to make it rain? Such questioning undoubtedly led man to endow the spirits with *patterns of behavior,* personality, motivation. When all these patterns were finally fitted together into a larger, all-embracing scheme, animism turned into religion, the spirits became gods. In this way an *order* of sorts was established in an otherwise incomprehensible universe. *Chaos* became *cosmos,* and the myths that were not made part of this new order became superstitions.

Around 600 B.C. in Greek Asia Minor, an idea emerged that was, as far as we know, without precedent. Thales, a Greek philosopher living in the Ionian town of Miletus, taught that the causes for the transformations we see in nature lie not so much in a world of spirits or gods, a world *apart* from the nature we observe, as in nature itself, particularly in that permanent aspect of nature we now call *matter*. This led to the births of *materialism, mechanism,* and *determinism.*

The propositions advanced by the pre-Socratic philosophers, Thales and his successors, at first merely tried to explain how seemingly profound changes could take place without the intervention of spiritual forces. Later, more detailed models were put forth. The earliest attempts were *monistic*: A single substance or principle was believed to account for all manifestations of matter. In this way changes were reduced to *changes in appearance* of the universal basic substance. By contrast, *pluralism*, which appeared somewhat later, explained the changeability of nature as the mixing and combining of a *number* of different basic substances. The assumption of a plurality of substances made possible the maintenance of constancy and permanence of every component in the mixture. The idea of a chemical element was born. But it was only in the *atomism* of Democritus (c. 460–370 B.C.) that the materialist-mechanist world picture reached its highest expression: All phenomena occurring in nature were ascribed to immutable, invisibly small grains of matter that were continuously in motion, not unlike our modern conception of the molecules of a gas. When the particles collided, each followed a precisely determined path. When they coalesced to form unions, the participating atoms were still there, buried in the compound and retrievable. Having always existed, they never had to be created, and they were absolutely indestructible. No power in the world, no spirit or god, was able to increase or diminish their number by a single one, or even deflect one from its inescapable trajectory.

Looking back on that relatively short period of natural philosophy between Thales and Democritus, we get the impression of a joyful, almost frenzied celebration of rational thought, as though man had just discovered his reasoning powers. Democritus called reason a delicate sense organ, much finer than those of sight and hearing, and the only source of true knowledge. "I would rather discover a single causal relationship," he said, "than be King of Persia."[5]

This peak of rationalist optimism was quickly abandoned in the subsequent Socratic and post-Socratic eras and was never again reached, not even in the most ebullient period of scientific triumphs toward the end of the nineteenth century. Of the scientific method John Burnet said that it represents thinking about nature "in the Greek way," and that a true scientific outlook—as distinguished from technological know-how—developed only among peoples who have come under the direct influence of the Greeks.[6] This is a sentiment many scientists find difficult to accept. The scientific method seems to them not only eminently reasonable; many believe that a thinking human really has no alternative. And yet Burnet's phrase suggests that science had to be *invented,* and that this happened not at the dawn of civilization but much later. Even more remarkable is the fact that science had such rough sledding for many centuries after that and is again under heavy assault.

What is the nature of the controversy and what are the competing patterns of thought? I mentioned the *order* that was created when animism became religion. Religion defined the relationship between man and the rest of the universe, described his origin and destiny, and prescribed patterns of behavior for every occasion. Mystery was not lifted from nature. Instead it was explained by a regression of mysterious causes—e.g., the world is held up by the shoulders of Atlas, who is standing on the back of a tortoise. The order created by this system was threatened only if you asked the wrong questions, such as "And what holds up the tortoise?" or "How do we know all this?" Thus the moral order established by religion was *intellectually chaotic.* By contrast, the natural philosophy of the pre-Socratics, in particular the atomic theory of Democritus, was a marvel of the intellect but a moral wasteland. There was no room for free will, hence no personal responsibility. In the last analysis there was only the eternal and inexorable motion of the atoms.

It is not surprising therefore that atomism became rejected, even despised, by later, more socially oriented Greek and Roman philosophers. Matter itself came to be regarded with contempt. This stigma persisted well into the seventeenth century when the physics of Galileo and Newton marked a return from the more adaptable Aristotelian principles to the hard-nosed materialism and determinism of the pre-Socratics.

There were, however, some attempts to ascribe mental functions to the physical brain long before the birth of physics in the seventeenth century. A few examples are given in the next chapter. With Galileo and Newton matter began to occupy once again the center of the intellectual stage, and it was taken for granted that matter was atomistic. The universe was viewed as a giant mechanism, and all its contents, including human brains, were likewise seen as mechanistic and deterministic systems. This viewpoint culminated in the materialism of eighteenth-century France.

Materialism began to undergo a change in the nineteenth century and has become relatively *soft* in the twentieth. The process started with the realization that physical systems composed of very large numbers of particles could not be treated *in practice* by a rigid application of the laws of mechanics derived by Newton. To describe the behavior of a gas, for example, it became necessary to admit our ignorance of microscopic details and to fill the gap with statistical arguments. *Statistical mechanics* thus lacks certainty *in practice*, even though the underlying mechanical laws would imply a certainty *in principle. If we could* determine the positions and the states of motion of every molecule in the gas, and *if we could* carry out the staggering volume of calculations necessary, then we *could in principle* predict what every molecule would do in the future. As it turns out, this hypothetical procedure may be impossible in *principle,* not just in practice. This is a point we will come back to in Chapter 6; it is an important point in assessing our ability or inability to determine the precise physical state of the brain.

The most profound changes in our conception of the physical universe came about in the twentieth century. The discovery of *quantum effects* by Planck, Einstein, Bohr, De Broglie, and others led to *quantum mechanics*, a radically new conception of matter and a description of the physical universe in which the classical passive observer is forced into active participation in the phenomena he is trying to describe. There has appeared also a new type of indeterminacy, or uncertainty of events, in addition to the classical uncertainties of statistical mechanics. I will discuss these indeterminacies in more detail in Chapter 6, together with a further source of uncertainty that has to do with a property called *self-reference*.

The old idea that matter consisted of immutable building blocks, the atoms or subunits of atoms, had to undergo a profound change also. John Dalton, the nineteenth-century British chemist who is generally considered to be the father of scientific atomism, still adhered to a philosophical notion that "all the changes we can produce, consist in separating particles that are in a state of cohesion or combination, and joining those that were previously at a distance."[7] This statement could have been made by Democritus over two millennia earlier.

But the particles of modern physics are very different from the atoms of Democritus or those of Dalton. Relativity has uncovered a strange connection between matter and space. The mass of the particle now depends on the velocity of the observer. The many transformations by which objects turn into other objects can no longer be interpreted as just the separation or the joining of elementary particles.

Matter has lost its ball-bearing hardness and the quality of immutable building blocks that had for so long been the very basis of physics. The search for the smallest units of matter that started so auspiciously with the dissection of the atom into electrons, protons, and neutrons, has led scientists into a labyrinth which shows little sign of being about to yield its secrets. Matter, the first aspect of nature to be demystified, today looms more mysteriously than ever, and Eddington's question, "What is it that haunts space where matter is found?" seems more appropriate than ever.

The transformations in our conceptions of matter have been slow to replace the old images. In the popular mind, matter has retained its aspect of simplicity to the point of dullness, of commonness to the point of vulgarity, and, to some, even its old Manichaean taint of evil. To explain any but the most transparent phenomenon in terms of matter and its interactions is often considered demeaning to the nobility of the phenomenon. This is particularly true when the phenomenon has to do with life, and the moreso the higher the form of life. The idealist may be criticized in many ways, but only his adversary, the materialist, is ever called *crass*.

How can we explain our aversion to the proposition that all the phenomena we associate with life will some day be derived from the properties of the matter of which our bodies are made? What accounts for the low regard some of us have for the material world?

Matter, when we look at its most elementary forms—protons, neutrons, electrons, plus a veritable zoo of exotic subnuclear particles, down to the elusive quarks—holds more than enough mystery to challenge the human intellect. On this strange stage, the stability of a feature means its persistence for periods as short as one hundred thousandth of a billionth of a billionth of a second, which is the time it takes a light ray to traverse the nucleus of an atom. Bulk matter may be more familiar to us, but it is really enormously more complex than a single elementary particle.

Now, take a system as exquisitely complex as the human body. Is there not enough *soul* in this structure to satisfy the most romantic view we have of ourselves? Why do we find it necessary to invoke metaphysics when we talk about life?

The answers to these questions are not difficult to find. The exquisiteness of our bodies does not hide from us the horror of their ultimate decay. We would do anything, believe almost anything, to make ourselves independent of these doomed vessels. And so we toss grappling hooks into the cosmos in the hope of gaining a permanent lifeline.

The prize we seek is always the same: consciousness away from our bodies. Almost anything will do. In Greek mythology the gloomy underworld of shadows was better than extinction. For the unrepentant Christian sinner, hell is the best *he* can hope for. For the Eastern mystic, the lifeline is some cosmic exhalation to which his consciousness can repair when his body fails, or even before. I submit that the cosmic connection we seek for mind and consciousness is the result of wishful thinking, and that we must look within the individual for a source of both.

Life can be said to have a *cosmic quality*. We believe now it can originate anywhere in the universe, given certain preconditions. Life is briefly held by individuals, but its main characteristics are transpersonal: It is passed on and it evolves. *Consciousness*, by contrast, is supremely personal. It begins when the first memories are laid down in the convolutions of the infant brain, and it deepens with the fashioning of a subjective world. It requires two things: a brain that is highly reflective, and a renewable, accessible store of memories. Neither of these appears to exist beyond the two ends of our life-span. We are born and we die unconscious.

The human as object

When we study any living thing, we begin with our knowledge of inanimate matter and see how far we can get. The physical complexity of even the simplest life-forms tends to obscure the question of whether the *substance* of life and the physical laws governing it are sufficient to account for life. In a sense, both the *physicalist*, who claims that they are sufficient, and the *vitalist,* who contends that they are not, are guessing at the outcome of that still-distant day when all *physical* processes taking place in living systems are thoroughly understood.

We can point with some pride to the progress we have made. We can describe the functions of most organs. Some we know so well that we are able to replace them, at least temporarily, with manmade machines: the heart, the lungs, and kidneys. We know much about the dynamics of muscle cells, neurons, and blood cells, and we have begun to understand the incredibly delicate mechanics of the genetic machinery. We understand some parts of the nervous system to be sequences of relays that pass signals from peripheral *sensors* to the central nervous system, and from there back to the periphery to control our muscles. We have at least the rudiments of an understanding of how the primitive earth several billion years ago cooked up the first prebiotic molecules from which all terrestrial life must have originated. And we can understand, in principle if not in detail, how the gigantic sweep of evolution follows from the double principle of chance mutation and Darwinian survival of the fittest. In all these investigations, no known physical law has been shown to be invalid, nor has it been demonstrated that any new laws peculiar to life have to be assumed.

When we turn our attention to human beings, the problem is exacerbated not so much by the fact that physical complexity is at its highest as by the emergence of a new world of phenomena that appears to lie outside the language and methodology we have developed for describing what we see around us.

The phenomena which are the source of all real knowledge are themselves mysterious. We call them *sensations*. It is possible and customary to circumvent the puzzle of sensations as long as the object of our study is part of the external world and thus is in the public domain. A simple example illustrates the point. Light of a certain wavelength (about 7000 angstroms, or one twenty-seven millionth of an inch) gives me the sensation I call *red*. This same light can be viewed by other persons. Although we cannot compare our sensations, we have agreed on the term *red* to denote the sensation, whatever it is, each of us registers when he views this light. The term *red* now denotes two things: my private sensation of redness and the occurrence of light of an agreed-upon physical quality (its wavelength). Note that the sensation itself may be different for each of us. It is necessary only that there be an internal consistency between my sensations and the physical stimuli causing them. For any individual the consistent pairing of his sensations, on the one hand, and physical qualities and events, on the other, is the single fact that puts him in touch with the world around him and at the same time gives meaning to talk about seeing red, feeling wind on one's face, or experiencing the mood of a sunset.

Most of the events behind our sensations are in the public domain. *Anyone* can feel the wind, see the sunset, etc. We can point them out. Thus when I talk about my sensations, the nature of the physical reality behind them is rarely in doubt, and the sensations themselves can be surmised by others from their own experiences of the same physical reality.

But not all sensations are caused by physical events that are in the public domain. We are often at a loss to describe the simple sensations coming from our own body sensors. In telling a physician how we are feeling, we may resort to synthetic descriptions like a "stabbing" pain, as though being stabbed were a common, shareable experience. In another situation an inarticulate "ecch" may be as descriptive of how we feel as any number of words.

The example of the patient-physician dialogue is apt, I think. The fundamental difficulty, the source of our frustration, has to do with the exclusiveness of sensations: Two people can look at the same star, but nobody has ever shared a headache.

Sensations are paired with stimuli, as observed above. But they are not constrained to follow, slavelike, the messages from our sensors, external or internal. We sometimes mistake the causes of sensations, and we manipulate sensations. While stimuli are impinging on our nervous system, we draw upon past experiences and project into the future. We even simulate events in our mind, often producing real sensations (just *imagine* someone scratching his fingernails across a blackboard). Finally, like Narcissus viewing his own image in the water, we can *reflect* upon our sensations, thereby changing them, and observe that change in an open-ended cycle that is perhaps the most characteristic feature of our mental activities.

Sensations are not just the end products of *sensory* processes—that is, the stimulation of *receptors*—they may also result from other neural or hormonal activity. I can have a sensation of being apprehensive, joyful, depressed, or sexually aroused.

A sensation that has significant ingredients of memory, projection into the future, and sensory or motor simulations, we call a *thought*. We thus erect a verbal structure around these phenomena and pretend that some identifiable physical reality is attached to them. We speak of being *shaken up* by one experience, *elated* by another, and of reacting to a third with *palpable fear.* According to one school of thought, the so-called *neural identity theory,* this is more than pretense. It is argued that definite physical states of the brain are to be *identified* with specific sensations. Furthermore, it is assumed that these *brain states,* although very complex, are *in principle* determinable. It would follow then that—once the identity between sensations and physical states of the brain was established—the privacy of the sensations would disappear, and sensations would be *reduced* to physical observables to be dealt with by the standard methods of physical science. This is the essence of *reductionism.* My sensations—from the simple sensation of *red* to the sensation of a mood, or the fleeting passage of a memory through my consciousness—would be in principle accessible to anyone equipped with what Donald McKay has called a *cerebroscope.*

Of course, as yet there is no such thing as a cerebroscope, and in later chapters I will argue that the idea such a device could some day be constructed is based on assumptions that are probably wrong. I believe that the privacy of sensations is inviolable, and if the physical scientist wishes to say anything about these phenomena, he must recognize the fundamental difference between observables that are in the common domain and the irrevocably private world of sensations.

It is somewhat puzzling that our attempts to give verbal expression to things we cannot point to has not been wholly unsuccessful. I deduce, by analogy with my own sensations, what *you* may sense when you say you feel lonely, happy, etc. But while my own sensations can never be in doubt, any statement I can make about your sensations remains conjecture. I can use such terms as *consciousness* or *will* or *mind,* and find that they will be understood in most contexts. At least, there seems to be agreement to accept them as conveying some meaning, even though there are schools of philosophy that say they have none. Still, consciousness cannot be measured or compared. Just like the sensations of which it is composed, it is private. This is probably why so many people believe they possess it in greater measure than others and offer to raise or at least alter that of their fellow humans. Paraphrasing Eddington, we may well ask, What is it that haunts matter where consciousness is found?

The last decade has seen a tremendous increase in public interest in matters of the mind. This consumer demand has led to a rash of literature on the subject, some of it novel and challenging but much of it of dubious value. Methods have been introduced that purport to be scientific but in effect have blurred the distinction between fact and fancy. As a result, the feeling has become widespread that not only is everything possible (nobody can argue with that), but everything is almost equally likely. To adopt that attitude is to give up hope of understanding anything, because understanding means that we consider some events more likely than others, some almost certain, and some very, very unlikely.

Remarks like mine are often met with complaints about scientific rigidity and with allegations of vested interests on the part of a scientific establishment. Past examples of great ideas nipped in the bud are always at hand. The scientific euphemism for such past errors is that the ideas had been "expressed before their time." Nor does it do any good to protest the scientist's evenhandedness and innovative spirit. Many scientists regard with suspicion opinions on science that originate outside of science, and their innovative spirit is often tempered by a strong conservative bent. Like nature itself, science embodies both continuity and change. It is forever maneuvering along a narrow line between dogma and gullibility. George Sarton, the great historian of science, remarked that:

> . . . to speak of the vested interests of science as one would of the vested interests of brewers or tobacco merchants is just as foolish as to speak of the vested interests of public health. When health officers have obtained good results at the cost of immense efforts, they will not permit any fool to jeopardize the lives of their community by untried expedients; the "vested interests" of astronomers, physicists, etc., are simply the interests of humanity.[8]

Sarton wrote these words in 1955, well past the age of innocence of science but a good decade before the onset of the great disillusionment. In 1969 Theodore Roszak spoke ominously of science or *technocracy* (he made no distinction between the two) leading to "an existence wholly estranged from everything that has ever made the life of man an interesting adventure."[9]

Practically all controversies in science revolve about the question of whether in a particular instance there is sufficient reason for making a break with a traditional line of approach, a set of principles, or theories, or whether one should continue in the same direction. Galileo had boldly accepted the new Copernican theory that removed the earth from the center of the universe, but he held on to the ancient notion of *epicycles* even though his contemporary, Kepler, provided him with powerful arguments to the contrary. Einstein never accepted some of the revolutionary premises of quantum mechanics, and more recently physicists have shown the greatest reluctance in giving up the cherished principle of left-right symmetry in nature.

With regard to mind and consciousness, there is no unanimity among scientists on whether any revisions are required in the body of science. There is in fact great uncertainty as to what if anything the scientist can do about these phenomena. Should we simply avoid the problem, noting that the objective of science is to make statements about collectively observable events, which excludes the domain of anyone's consciousness? We could—except for the fact that these consciousnesses have a habit of intruding upon and changing events in the world we *do* observe collectively.

Vernon Reynolds, in his book *The Biology of Human Action*, argues against the tendency of some anthropologists to *biologize* their science; that is, to deduce human actions from their biological substrate—our genetic makeup and the neural machinery: "In the last analysis, it is what we *think* that counts . . . the conceptual mind that sets us apart from other species."[10] Can we then somehow include our thoughts in the dynamics of the body? Are thoughts in turn reducible to sets of stimuli, past and present, that are processed through our internal neuronal and hormonal computers?

The answers to these questions are not easy to come by. It will be necessary to take a very careful look at the brain, the system through which all these processes pass, and at the processes themselves as far as they can be identified. The *machine* has been a most helpful metaphor when studying the functioning of various parts of the body. In the brain, too, we speak of *mechanisms* by which certain functions are accomplished. But the machine-body analogy breaks down, I believe, in certain significant respects that concern the unassailable individuality of humans. This includes such features as an intrinsic unpredictability and the impossibility to duplicate or reset. Unlike a computer, which can be made to yield all its stored information (by printing and transferring it to some other memory device or to another computer), no human can willingly or unwillingly be drained of all his knowledge.

There is no transfer of information between humans that corresponds to what in computer jargon is called a "dump," that is, the unconditional release of *all* stored information.

Man's fear of the void applies more than anything else to his own knowledge. The failure of science to provide a clear approach to questions touching on our minds has left a gap we are only too eager to fill with intuition or fantasy. In the seventies this led to an almost compulsive preoccupation with the *self*, a massive assault on the mind reminiscent of previous concerted efforts to unlock the atom or to put a man on the moon. But unlike those efforts, which were carried out by relatively small, very coherent, single-minded groups, the *mind project* has the character of a happening in which the achievement of specific goals has become secondary to *doing your own thing*.

This unprecedented ferment has caused both excitement among some onlookers and despair among others. There is the feeling among those in the first group that we have at last freed ourselves from the constraints of rational thought (*linear thinking* is the pejorative term often used), and that ours is an intoxicating age of great and profound revelations.

Seen from a different perspective, the arena appears to be populated by a strange troupe of mountebanks, popping in and out of their own bodies at will and bending keys with their minds, and gurus exploding consciousnesses like so many balloons. The second group of onlookers lament the abandonment of rigid criteria for truth and the antiscientific character of the goings-on. They are convinced that, the massive participation notwithstanding, little of enduring value will emerge.

It would be wrong to suggest that scientists invariably belong to the latter disenchanted group. In the fabric of science, particularly in twentieth-century physics, there has been more than a thread of mysticism. Many leading theoretical physicists have shown a tendency to link up with doctrines lying outside the body of established facts. To varying degrees many, but probably a minority of scientists, would contend that there is a value to knowledge irrationally acquired and a validity to physical events defying physical laws. In particular, many feel that the puzzles of mind and consciousness demand both a relaxation of the rigid standards imposed by science and the application of extrascientific methods.

My description of the two distinct groups of spectators is thus an oversimplification. Compulsive classifiers have been put in their place once and for all by the statement that "there are only two kinds of people: those who divide all of humanity into two categories, and those who don't." What is really unfolding before us is an intellectual drama that may become the play of the century. It deals with the assault on what has been called the last frontier of knowledge, man's brain and mind, and the relation between the two: the world knot.

Outline

Before the scope of this book becomes too extravagant, I would like to outline the topics that look attractive and manageable as seen from this panoramic view, and then approach the subject matter.

We will begin with a discussion of the human nervous system. An enormous amount of new knowledge has been gathered about our brains in the last few decades, and Chapters 2, 3, and 4 will attempt to present some of the basic structural and functional properties as they are now recognized. We will also take a look at some of the major controversies that still dominate the field. We will be concerned with the manner in which information about the world is picked up by our delicate senses, and how, starting from the day we are born, these messages are filtered, coded, and transformed by our nervous system and enter the windows of the mind.

But we shall not stop there because it is at this point that the most vital questions concerning our true nature present themselves. Machines can be equipped with delicate sensors and can be made to perform the most complex tasks. Are we then anything more than very exquisite machines?

"Nothing more," says the classical materialist.

"But I have consciousness," you will say, "and I feel pain and pleasure."

"Tell me precisely what you mean by this, and I will build you a machine with what you call consciousness and feelings," answers the reductionist.

These are classic arguments, and they have been all but exhausted. Do we have anywhere else to go? It has been suggested that, as in the case of black holes in astronomy and quarks in the physics of elementary particles, we may have reached the end of what is knowable. Why then go on with this inquiry?

There are several reasons. The limits of knowledge set by the most visionary of men have in the end always been transcended. We simply don't know what the true limits are. In the case of the problems at hand there have lately been numerous unexpected advances. Our understanding of perception has deepened significantly, as I will try to show in Chapter 5, in which I will also discuss some recent experiments that may alter our thinking about consciousness and free will.

In seeming contradiction to the preceding paragraph, Chapter 6 will talk about some limits to our knowledge. Returning once again to the *mechanisms* that operate in our nervous system, we realize that they are of a unique kind. The brain is a *macroscopic* system, but *microscopic* states, such as the firings of individual neurons and phenomena on even smaller scales, play decisive roles. For all we know, the only meaningful description of the *state of the brain* would have to include the complete specifications of *which* of the billions of neurons are firing at this moment, and the next, and the next.

But here we find ourselves confronted with certain seemingly unsurmountable limitations, which are not due to ignorance or lack of vision on our part but, on the contrary, to new insights into the nature of things. Indeterminacies and uncertainties arise from the intrinsically statistical nature of the macrocosm. An additional indeterminacy may come from the property of self-reference possessed by the conscious, reasoning brain.

After these excursions into the realms of chance and uncertainty, we will reconsider in Chapter 7 the classical problem of the relation between body and mind. I will argue that the above considerations raise serious doubts about any theory that involves the predictions, determinations, and interpretations of *detailed* states of the nervous system. This applies, for example, to the *psychophysical identity theory*, which asserts that such physical states are *identical* to particular psychological or mental states. We encountered an extreme form of this in J. Z. Young's statement quoted earlier.

But I find dualism an equally unacceptable alternative. It confounds the problem and explains nothing. In Chapter 7 I will try to put together a point of view which I believe to be compatible with the theoretical and empirical facts as presented here. We will also take a look again at the analogy between man and machine. Since there is no machine like man, what we are really asking is whether, in principle, such a machine could be built. The words "in principle" are decisive here. The answer can be "yes" only if no known principles are violated. On the basis of what we will have discussed in Chapter 6, we will offer a cautious "maybe, but probably no."

It is tempting for a scientist to believe that the scientific approach to problems is not just the only rational one but that it is also the *natural* one. This would imply that there is something in the way we human beings think which causes us to proceed along rational lines.

Such, however, is not the case. Science, or rather the mental habits and attitudes from which science arose, was *invented* by Greek philosophers some 2600 years ago. We know of no earlier examples of this particular approach to the problems of nature. And notwithstanding the spectacular successes of the method, it has never completely replaced earlier thinking patterns. Religions and other forms of mysticism are still with us. This is very puzzling, even disturbing to many scientists, but it, too, is a fact. I say this not to propose an egalitarian theory of knowledge but merely to dispel the notion that science is the *natural* way of thinking about nature. I do believe it is the *correct* way.

Why the disparity of human thought persists is a curious fact that says not so much about nature as about *human nature*. But until the full meaning of this message is understood, we have only partial knowledge of what it is to be human.

I have added an epilogue (Chapter 8), in which I relate some personal experiences that predate by many years my professional involvement with the human brain. The events illustrate the point made above, but I don't pretend to understand all the implications. It is perhaps appropriate to end on this note of uncertainty.

2

CLOSEUP:
THE BRAIN
FROM THE TOP

Oh the nerves, the nerves; the mysteries of this machine called Man! Oh the little that unhinges it: poor creatures that we are!

—CHARLES DICKENS, The Chimes. Third Quarter

We begin with a short look at some early ideas about the human brain. These are instructive because some of the conflicting views that have persisted to this day have a long history. Also the twin problems of *structure* and *function* appear inseparable right from the start, like the two faces of a coin.

We will learn about neurons and their mode of operation. Neurons are the tiny units from which all nervous tissue is constructed. They communicate with one another by electrical signals sent along microscopic fibers that connect them in chains and networks that stretch from the surface of the body, where they are in touch with the outside world, to the brain and back to the surface of the body. We will follow these chains of messengers rapidly to the place where everything seems to happen: the *neocortex* of the brain. Like impatient explorers, having bypassed the so-called lower centers, we will now look for the highest pinnacle, the command center, the ultimate authority. We won't find it and will conclude there probably is no such thing.

Later, in Chapter 4, we will go back to the more peripheral structures in search of the real meaning of neural activity. We will then return to questions about the neural nature of such things as sensations, consciousness, and the mind.

The synthesis which I hope will emerge from all this will not be so much a matter of new ideas as a juxtaposition of facts gathered from the neurosciences and from physics, which still has the last word about what we can and cannot expect from physical systems.

The two concepts, structure and function, are the pillars of biology. When we contemplate any living system, or part of it, we generally ask, "What does it look like?" and "What does it do?" These two questions don't exactly exhaust all our curiosity about the creature or the organ. We may also wish to know how it evolved, what are its principal malfunctions, and how they may be overcome. But with a knowledge of the structure and a good understanding of its mode of operation we have not only satisfied most of our curiosity, we have also made a good start toward answering all the other questions we might raise.

The mammalian brain represents the ultimate in structural complexity. Nowhere in the explored universe do we know of a system that is as intricate and whose functioning is more obscure than the 1400 grams of human brain. In one other respect are its structure and function unique. The exposed brain is the most vulnerable tissue in the body. It has the consistency of a paste. The slightest pressure in some places can cause lethal damage. A freshly excised human brain laid on a flat surface would most likely distort and rupture under its own weight. On the other hand, substantial damage to brain tissue caused by accidents or disease sometimes produces functional changes that are relatively minor. There is a classic case in the annals of medicine. In 1848 Phineas Gage, a construction worker in Cavendish, Vermont, suffered massive brain damage when a heavy steel rod was driven through his skull during a blasting operation. He survived but with a very different personality. Efficient and likable before the accident, he now became shiftless and abusive. Still, considering the frightful destruction in his head, his survival seems miraculous. This combination of structural delicacy and functional ruggedness constitutes one of the many puzzling aspects of the brain.

Early ideas: antiquity through the Renaissance

It has not always been recognized that the brain is the seat of our mental activities. The Homeric heroes *thought* in their bellies, specifically their diaphragms. As early as the fifth century B.C., Alcmaeon of Croton and Hippocrates had ascribed all emotional activities and mental faculties to the brain. But later Aristotle believed the heart to be the center of the nervous system.

Knowledge progressed with painful slowness. Six centuries after Hippocrates, another Greek physician, Galen (c. A.D. 130–200), studied the sensory pathways that lead to the brain, the *"way in,"* as Sir Charles Sherrington called it much later. Galen's knowledge of anatomy was gained from dissections he performed on apes and pigs. In all probability, no human cadavers were used for study at that time. Galen again correctly identified the brain as the nervous center and described the nerve bundles that emanate from the peripheral sense organs, such as the eyes, as *conductors* for sensory information to the brain. He puzzled much over the nature of the flow of signals, coming to the conclusion finally that an invisible fluid, or *pneuma,* was transported through these nerves and was responsible also for activity in the brain itself. It was probably this notion of a *fluid* constituting mental activity that for many centuries after Galen caused anatomists to pay more attention to the *cavities* in the brain, the so-called cerebral *ventricles,* than to the brain itself.

Progress could come only from direct observation of the internal human anatomy. This meant dissection of human cadavers. Such activity had to overcome powerful taboos and a natural revulsion against manipulating the dead. Human dissections were carried out at the University of Bologna as early as A.D. 1200, and perhaps even earlier in Salerno, just south of Naples, where the medical school dates back to the ninth century.

The success of the School of Salerno derived from the heterogeneity of its faculty. We could think of it as the first school in which affirmative action was practiced. Among the minorities holding teaching positions were Greeks, Jews, and Saracens. Some of the professors teaching medicine were women. Here for the first time, knowledge from widely differing cultural backgrounds was pooled, and the Western world became reacquainted with early Greek scholarship, which the Arabs had learned from Greeks in the Byzantine Empire.

To the School of Salerno must therefore go the credit for reestablishing a learned tradition in Western medicine, which in the earlier Middle Ages had largely been reduced to folklore and superstition.

The Catholic Church did not look with favor upon such practice of human dissection and did not officially sanction it until quite late. In

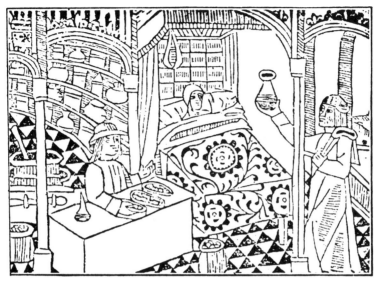

2.1 *Doctor, patient, and chemist at the School of Salerno*

the anatomy theater built at the University of Bologna in 1637, an inquisitor could at all times observe the proceedings through a small window from an adjoining room and could interrupt the anatomist's lecture with spiritual comments. Even so, two parts of the human body were supposed to be excluded from examination: the sex organs and the brain.

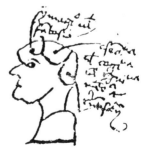

2.2 *Sketch, dated 1413, showing three human brain functions, in* Cod. lat. Monacensis. *(From Sudhoff)*

In a sketch dated 1413 (Fig. 2.2) an unknown anatomist indicated the regions he considered responsible for the three brain functions. Translated from the barely legible Latin, these are from front to back: "imagination or fantasy," "guessing or thinking," and "memory or *common sense.*" It was believed that all the sensory inputs to the brain converged at a single *common* location, the *sensus communis.* Although the meaning has changed, the expression *common sense* is undoubtedly derived from that term.

The idea of three distinct brain functions was expressed again about a hundred years later by the Carthusian monk Gregor Reisch in a sketch showing three prominent ventricles, or brain cavities (Fig. 2.3). Here the labels are *sensus communis, fantasia, imaginativa; cogitativa, estimativa,* and *memorativa.* Sensory information from the eye,

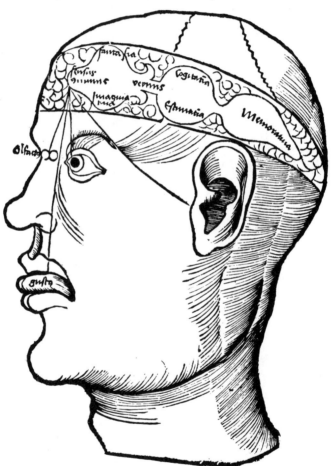

2.3 *Brain functions according to Gregor Reisch (c.* A.D. *1467–1525). This is an example of the* cell theory *according to which the prominent brain cavities, or* ventricles, *have specific cognitive functions. The senses of sight, hearing, smell, and taste are seen to converge on the first cell containing the* sensus communis. (*In* Margarita Philosophica, *G. Reisch, Heidelberg, 1504*)

ear, tongue, and nose is *seen* to *converge* at the *common sense* at the front of the brain. From there it apparently *flows* through the central cavity (thinking) and winds up as memory in the last ventricle. The narrow passage between the first and second compartments is labeled *vermis,* Latin for worm. It was later believed to act as a valve controlling the flow of information into the thinking compartment, thus turning thought on and off. Reisch's drawing was often copied and was to have a profound and lasting effect on subsequent ideas about brain function.

Early anatomical dissections proceeded in a peculiar manner. The lecturer, sitting on a rostrum, read from a prepared text, rarely looking down at the dissection, which was performed by an assistant (Fig. 2.4). In 1543 Andreas Vesalius described an anatomy lecture as:

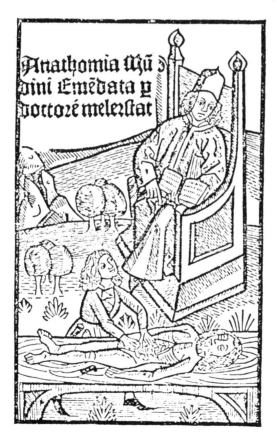

2.4 *Anatomy lesson.(In* Anatomy *of Mundinus Melerstat edition,Leipzig, c. 1493)*

> . . . a detestable ceremony in which certain persons are accustomed to perform a dissection of the human body while others narrate the history of the parts: these latter from a lofty pulpit and with egregious arrogance sing like magpies of things whereof they have no experience . . .[1]

Unlike their academic contemporaries, many Renaissance painters learned their anatomy firsthand from dissections performed on animals and humans. Leonardo da Vinci tells us of "the fear of passing the night hours in the company of these corpses, quartered and flayed and horrible to behold."[2]

Still, the brain eludes Leonardo's meticulous eye and appears strangely primitive (Fig. 2.5) when we compare it with his other anatomical sketches. It is almost as though he were heeding a last taboo: not to look under the human skull. Actually we know from his accounts that he had done many dissections of the brain, but, following the prejudices of his time, he was mainly interested in one feature he could not *dissect out*—the ventricles. Contrast this with the realistic and painstaking engraving of the brain by Vesalius (Fig. 2.6).

No one has influenced thinking about mind and brain more lastingly than the French mathematician, philosopher, and scientist René Descartes. It is said that Descartes spent some seven years in Leiden dissecting brains and eyes. He was convinced that the human body was a *machine* that could be understood completely through physical laws. This applied also to the brain, except that it was inhabited by a nonmaterial entity, the *soul*. The machine-like brain and the soul, according to Descartes, interacted at the pineal body, a small, cone-shaped gland of unknown function in the third ventricle.

Medieval notions about the relationship between brain and mind are reflected in the treatment of mental diseases. The practice of admitting mental cases to hospitals goes back at least to the beginning of the thirteenth century and attests to an early recognition of a physical basis for mental phenomena. By the end of the thirteenth century some hospitals had already specialized in mental diseases; London's Bedlam Hospital was perhaps the best known among them. It was believed that there were three possible causes for these disorders: physical, mental, and spiritual. To the first category belonged such afflictions as rabies and alcoholism; to the second, melancholy. The spiritual causes generally meant some form of demonic possession. This is in accordance with an ancient belief in the supernatural origin of mental diseases.

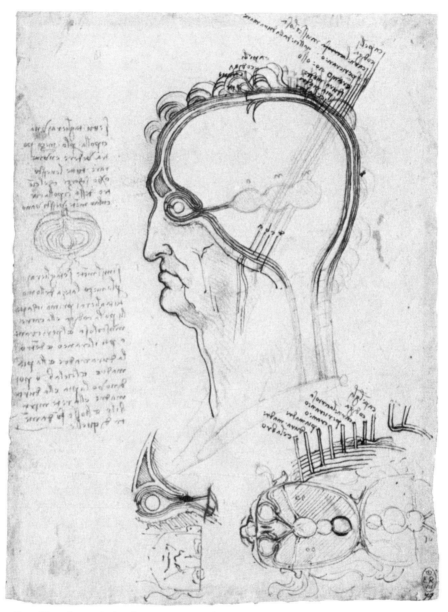

2.5 *Sketches of the human brain by Leonardo da Vinci. (Royal Library of Windsor)*

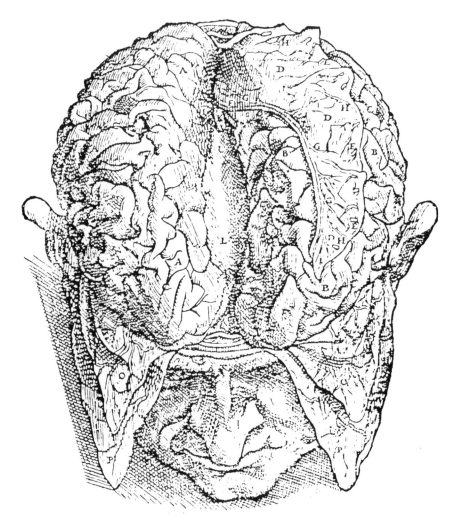

2.6 *Etching of the brain by Vesalius* (Seventh Book on Anatomy)

Treatments for this last category were designed to annoy and eventually drive out the demon. Their noxious effects on the patient were considered to be of minor importance. It was even believed that the possessed person had no sensation, that any discomfort or pain inflicted was felt only by the demon, not by the patient. These notions, and their survival in various forms almost to this day, were undoubtedly sustained by the fact that amnesias often accompany fits and seizures. Thus the person returning to a normal state of mind often has no recollection of the pains and terrors he has experienced. The Church, of course, considered any form of demonic possession to be within its competence and jurisdiction. "The exorcist," says an old manual of exorcism, "is not only a minister of the Church, but he is also a doctor of souls."

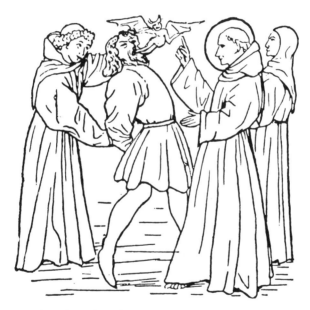

2.7 *A medieval saint exorcizing a demon*

Neurons:
the way in and the way out

The preceding section is not just of historical interest. I included it to bring out the fact that in our present reflections on the mind-body problem, we are only going over ground that has been worked for a long time. Current attempts to read meaning into the electrical activities of neurons are perhaps not so far removed from Galen's theory of an invisible fluid flowing through nerve fibers. By this I don't mean to belittle current scientific theory or to lend undue weight to primitive notions of the past. We gain, I believe, a valuable perspective from the realization that we are always limited by the available repertoire of physical concepts when we try to find mechanisms for life functions.

In this section we pick up the story of the structure and function of the brain at our present level of knowledge.

The human central nervous system consists of the brain and the spinal cord. From these two structures radiates a system of fibers, really bundles of fibers, that branch and fan out to all other parts of the body. These fibers are the *nerves*. Contrary to some popular notions, as expressed by the phrase "It's just nerves," nerves are real and material, just like flesh and sinew and bone. They are *cables* that carry signals to or from the central nervous system, as Galen realized long ago. We now know the nature of these signals, their origin and destination. But, first, a little more about the overall plan.

The nerves are one-way paths; they go from one part of the body to another. In the traditional picture of the nervous system, they either come from *sensors* or they go to *effectors*. That is, they either gather information from sense organs—the eyes, the ears, the skin senses, the internal senses—and conduct them to the brain; or they take *instructions* from the central nervous system to the muscles and glands they control. The first system is also called the *afferent* system, the one that gathers and brings in information: the second is the *efferent* system, the one that goes out, controls, issues commands. The English physiologist, Sir Charles Sherrington (1857–1952), who pioneered much of modern neuroscience, spoke of the two systems as "the way in" and "the way out."

The efferent system can be further divided into one system of voluntary control and one of *autonomic* control. The muscles that move our arms and fingers, and all other *skeletal* muscles, are under the control of the voluntary motor system, while heartbeat and respiration are part of the autonomic system. An understanding of the brain is further complicated by its many other *silent* functions: the regulation of the body's chemistry through control over the master gland, the *pituitary*, and the regulation of vital variables such as body temperature, blood pressure, and others. We will be concerned mainly with the brain's sensory and voluntary motor functions.

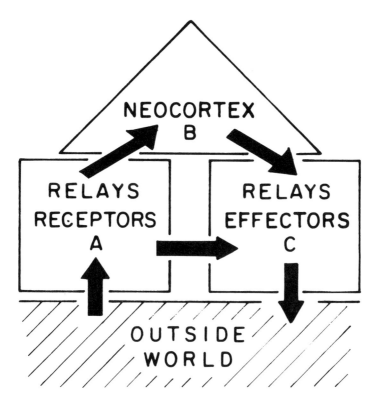

2.8 *An overview of the nervous system*

With this restriction I have sketched in Fig. 2.8 a very general schematic plan. The nervous system is represented by three units that communicate with the environment, the shaded area below. The box on the left (A) represents the various sensors and the peripheral pathways and relays. This part is the afferent or *ascending* portion of the nervous system. On the right of the diagram (C) we have the *descending* portion, pathways that lead down from the brain to the motor system, the *effectors*, which act on the outside world through the body's muscles. Prominent among the afferent pathways is the optic nerve, a bundle of about a million tiny fibers that run from each eye to the brain. On the efferent side is the so-called *pyramidal tract*, a cable that descends from the brain into the spinal cord, then branches out to contact all the voluntary muscles in our body.

The pyramid (B), sitting on top of the whole structure in Fig. 2.8, is the *highest* portion of the *brain*, the *cerebral cortex*. It is kept informed about the world by the afferent fibers and issues orders through the descending, or efferent, fibers.

The overall plan of Fig. 2.8 stresses the *up-down* character of the organization of the nervous system: *Up* is away from the receptors and toward the brain, *down* is away from the brain and toward the effectors.

The arrow going directly from (A) to (C) represents *reflexes*. These are pathways allowing certain stimuli to activate muscle action directly; that is, without intervention by higher brain centers.

By drawing the cortex itself in the shape of a pyramid, we express the often-held view that the highest structure shares this up-down directionality with the rest of the nervous system. This raises the question of where the uppermost portion of the brain can be found. We will return to this point in Chapter 3.

All parts of the nervous system are connected internally and with one another by *nerves*. But their significance must not be exaggerated. They are the cables, the arrows in Fig 2.8, that *transport* information; they neither generate it nor act on it. They make no decisions. For these functions we have to look at what goes on at either end of these cables.

But before we do that we must learn about the fundamental structural and functional unit of any nervous system, the *neuron*. We owe the concept of individual neurons to the great Spanish anatomist Santiago Ramón y Cajal (1852–1934). Cajal was among the first to realize that the nervous systems of all animals and of man consist of many individual cells that are quite distinct from each other, but communicate with one another at special locations called *synapses*. Neurons come in many sizes and shapes, but there are a few important things they all have in common.

> 1. A neuron is a living cell. Unlike most other cells, which are compact in shape, the neuron generally has a number of processes or fibers extending from the main body of the cell, sometimes branching profusely and reaching out over considerable distances. These are, however, part of that cell; a single continuous membrane covers the cell body and all its projections.
>
> 2. The neuron membrane is *excitable*. An important feature that distinguishes the neuron from most other cells is that the membrane is specialized to carry electrical signals which travel *to* the cell body along some fibers and *away* from it on others. Later

we will be more specific about these signals and their mode of travel.

3. Neurons are links in a network. They generally receive information *from*, and pass information on *to* other neurons. I say *generally* because there are two exceptions: *Receptors* are neurons that are stimulated directly by the environment: the photoreceptors in the eye by light, the touch receptors in the skin by pressure. Receptors transmit their signals to other neurons. On the other hand, *effectors* receive their signals from other neurons but act directly on muscles or glands and thus affect the environment. "Environment" here means anything that is not neurons. A touch receptor at the fingertip and a pain receptor in the gut both *sense* the environment.

4. Neurons pass information to other neurons through specialized junctions called *synapses*. These structures are extremely small and can be seen only with the aid of an electron microscope.

The above characteristics are shared by all neurons. We will take a look now at the most common type of neuron found in the mammalian nervous system. Such a *typical* neuron is shown in Fig. 2.9. It has three distinct parts: a cell body or soma; a set of branching fibers called *dendrites*; and a single branching fiber called the *axon*. The dendrites are often distinguished by the fact that they have a *hairy* appearance under the microscope. The little projections are called *spines*. Each spine is in fact the site of a synapse; that is, a point at which another neuron makes a junction with this neuron. A single neuron may have thousands of spines, each a location where signals enter from other parts of the nervous system. The function of the dendrite is to gather these signals and to conduct them to the cell body, where they are added together.

Unlike the dendrites, the axon is a *single* smooth fiber that also branches out and sometimes travels a considerable distance away from the cell body. The *response* of the cell to all the incoming signals is carried by the axon and transported away from the cell body and *to* the junctions or synapses the cell makes with other cells.

At this point, it is important that we know something more about the nature of the signals which come in on the dendrites and exit along the axon. First, take a look at the dendrites: The cell membrane envelops all the cell processes. A piece of dendrite therefore is like a sec-

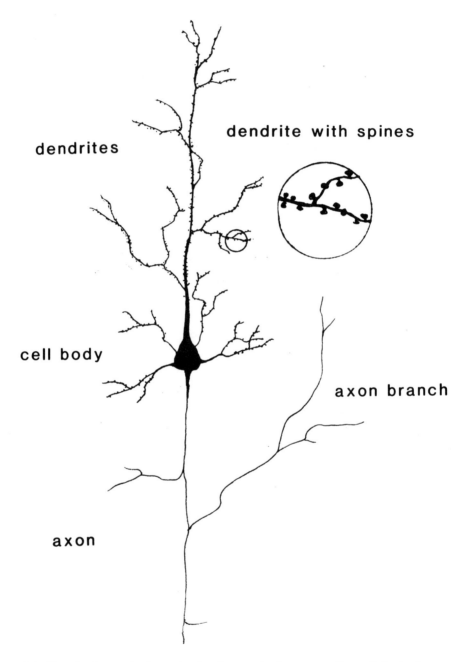

2.9 *Sketch of a typical neuron in the cerebral cortex. The cell body has a pyramidal shape, and the branching dendrites are covered with* spines. *The axon is smooth but also branches.*

tion of a garden hose which, instead of water, contains part of the cytoplasm or intracellular fluid. The outside of the wall is bathed in the extracellular fluid that fills the space between cells. It is the nature of the wall and of these two different fluids that there will normally be a difference of *electric potential* between the inside and the outside, very much like the voltage that appears between the terminals of a battery. But whereas in a common automobile battery the potential difference is about twelve volts, it is somewhat less than one tenth of a volt in the case of a cell membrane. This is called the *resting potential.* When resting, the outside of the membrane is positive with respect to the inside.

A signal coming in on one of the spines changes these electrical properties; it increases or decreases the positivity of the outside of the membrane. We speak in the first case of a *hyperpolarization,* in the second of a *depolarization* of the dendritic wall. It is the nature of an excitable membrane that such a local disturbance does not remain stationary but travels along the fiber very much like the snap of a whip or a kink in a stretched rope.

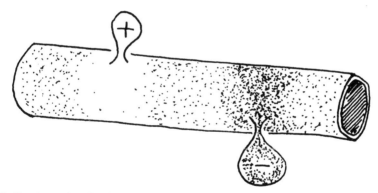

2.10 *Section of a dendrite with two spines. Dark shading at the right indicates a pulse of depolarization traveling along the surface. Also an inhibitory postsynaptic potential (hyperpolarization) is shown starting at the spine on the left.*

Figure 2.10 shows a short section of a dendrite. Its negative interior is shown in black, the outside of its membrane in gray, where it is in the resting state. The dark ring near the right end represents a region that is less positive than resting, hence it is *depolarized.* Farther to the left is a light-colored region where the potential is higher than normal.

This is a *hyperpolarized* region. These electric disturbances, called *postsynaptic potentials*, travel rapidly along the dendrites.

The dendritic trees of a neuron can be pictured as gatherers of signals, some positive and some negative. All these signals are funneled down the dendrites toward the cell body, where they are all added up. The actual membrane potential at the part of the cell body where the axon begins is crucial in what happens next. This potential will determine whether or not the cell responds with an *action potential* to all the signals it has received. For this to happen, the membrane potential in that region must be reduced, that is depolarized, below a certain critical value called the *threshold*. For that reason depolarizing potentials are called *excitatory*. Hyperpolarizing signals take the membrane away from the threshold and are therefore called *inhibitory*.

The signals that travel out along the axon are also electric. For most neurons they are called *action potentials* and differ from the postsynaptic potentials on the dendrites in several important respects. There is only one type of action potential. Whereas postsynaptic potentials come in all sizes and two polarities, the action potential is a standard electric *spike* of about one tenth of a volt in height. It is produced at the beginning of the axon whenever the membrane potential at that point has dropped below the threshold. From there the action potential travels rapidly, and without getting any weaker, toward the axon endings. Because of these features, we speak of the *all-or-none* response of the cell. The propagation of the spike along the axon can be compared with a traveling smoke ring. It is a vortex of electric current that propels itself along the fiber and gets steadily reinforced as it progresses.

There remains one gap in this picture; it is quite literally a *gap*. Along its way each axon contacts many of the *synapses*. Here the action potentials of one cell produce the postsynaptic potentials on other cells. Synapses are incredibly delicate structures, still far from completely understood. Also there are many different types of synapses, which are so complex and varied that a whole branch of neuroscience, called *synaptology*, is devoted to their study. I will briefly describe one type only.

A type of synapse often encountered in the brain is shown in Fig. 2.11. In this schematic drawing, the end of an axon coming in from the upper right partly envelops one of the spines of the dendrite of another cell. Note that a narrow gap is left between the membranes. At the axon side of the synaptic junction, electron micrographs reveal tiny

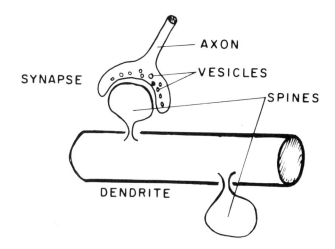

2.11 *Schematic drawing of an axon ending making a synapse on the spine of a dendrite. Note the narrow gap between the two cell membranes.*

spherical bubbles called *synaptic vesicles.* These are filled with a special chemical called a *transmitter substance.* When an action potential arrives at the axon terminal, these vesicles release their cargo of transmitter molecules into the synaptic gap. The molecules then cross the gap and attach themselves to the membrane of the dendritic spine.

There are many different types of transmitter molecules, but they all have the property of changing the potential of the cell membrane on which they land, providing the membrane has receptor sites which are specific for the molecules. It appears now that the family of these chemical messengers in the brain is much larger than was previously believed. They not only act locally across the synaptic gaps, but some of them may be carried to more distant locations by the bloodstream or by the cerebrospinal fluid. We can think of these molecules as forming an information-carrying network that is superimposed on the more locally acting neural system. If this long-range chemical information exchange turns out to have the significance many scientists presently attribute to it, it represents a curious return to the ancient notion of information coursing through the ventricles of the brain. At the end of Chapter 4 we will discuss some of these new findings in brain chemistry.

For the moment we are more concerned with what happens at specific synapses. The transmitter molecules released by the vesicles of the axon will cause the membrane-potential changes at the dendrites: toward the threshold when they are excitatory, away from the threshold when they are inhibitory.

Let us now recapitulate briefly the whole chain of events that takes place in a network of neurons. Start with a neuron that has just *fired*, that is, has produced an action potential. This electric pulse travels down the axon of the cell and all its branches. When it reaches a synapse, it causes the release of a transmitter substance which in turn causes the dendritic membrane potential to change. Each neuron receives such signals from many other neurons. These messages are continuously flowing down the dendrites to the cell body, where they are mixed and added. If, as a result, the membrane potential drops below the threshold at any time, *that* cell too will fire. As long as the threshold is not reached, the cell remains silent. The time taken between the firing of one cell and the responsive firing of another cell is a few thousandths of a second.

The next diagram (Fig. 2.12) shows a minute portion of a network of neurons. At the upper left the axon from cell A (cell body not shown) makes a synapse on a dendrite of neuron B (the cell body and parts of its many dendrites are shown). We also see a portion of the axon of neuron B, one branch of which makes a synapse on the dendrite of a third neuron, C.

The almost featureless lump of approximately ten billion neurons in our brain—which someone has likened to a "bowlful of porridge"— now takes on a new aspect. We see a vast network of cells talking to one another in the language of tiny electrical blips, the action potentials. These blips are *heard* by other cells as postsynaptic potentials, and the answer is another blip—or silence. This is called the all-or-none response.

Logic of impoverished neurons

The forties and fifties were a yeasty time, full of excitement and promise in the sciences. The age of the first electronic computers began around 1943 and straddled the end of World War II, from which it took much of its impetus. In rapid succession such electronic behemoths as the ENIAC, the UNIVAC, and MIT's Whirlwind computer made their appearance, only to be replaced by machines that were more sophisticated, faster, and, in general, smaller. Three innova-

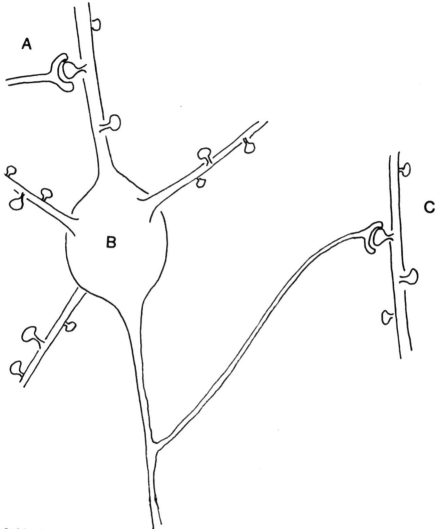

2.12 *An axon from neuron A makes a synaptic contact with a dendrite of a second neuron B, whose axon, in turn, synapses on a dendrite of a third neuron, C.*

tions were primarily responsible for the spectacular advancements: the storing of instructions, or *programs*, in the computer's own memory; the use of binary, or two-valued, logic; and the replacement of bulky vacuum tubes by transistors.

Behind many of the developments in computer design was the brilliant Hungarian-born physicist and mathematician John von Neumann. It was inevitable that sooner or later the logical power of these new devices should be compared to that of human brains, and von Neumann was one of the first to discuss this subject in detail.[3] Such analogies were especially tempting, because the brain too apparently has the programs for its operation stored in its own memory banks, and its units employ a kind of binary logic: A neuron either fires an action potential or it doesn't.

Intrigued with their own creations, scientists began to speculate—and are still speculating—just how far computers might go toward imitating and perhaps replacing human intelligence. Can computers think? Can computers feel? Will computers take over?

It became obvious at the same time that there remained some significant differences. Social scientists who have tried to simulate human affairs by the use of computers have pointed out that human folly is often more difficult to simulate than human intelligence. It is necessary, for example, to restrict severely the computer's ability to predict the future if one wants it to commit the equivalent of a warlike act. Norbert Wiener wrote in 1963 in the introduction to a Symposium on Nerve, Brain, and Memory Models:

> In a comparative study of human performance and machine performance, it must be realized that the human being does some things much better than the machine and some things worse. The human system is not as precise nor as quick as a computing machine. On the other hand, the computing machine tends to go to pieces unless all details of its programming are strictly determined. The human being has a great capacity for achieving results while working with imperfect programming. We can do a tremendous amount with vague ideas, but to most existing machines vague ideas are of absolutely no use.[4]

Norbert Wiener had been engaged at that time in a scientific revolution of his own. Apart from his many contributions in pure and applied mathematics, he introduced in 1948 a new concept and a new field of study: *cybernetics*. This was a general theory of control devices in which the engineering principle of feedback is used to obtain certain desired conditions. Its prototype is the governor on a steam engine, which is activated by excessive pressure in the boiler to release steam and which shuts off automatically when the pressure has dropped to normal.

The principle of the governor can be extended to more sophisticated control devices and even to biological processes, such as the regulation of body temperature and metabolic functions, and—more generally—to the maintenance of an organism's well-being in a hostile and hazardous environment. It is natural to think of the functioning of the brain in terms of such cybernetic principles. This approach was pioneered by Warren McCulloch at MIT, who as early as 1943 published a paper with Walter Pitts entitled "A Logical Calculus of the Ideas Immanent in Nervous Activity."[5] This paper has had an enormous influence on subsequent brain theories, since it demonstrated the virtually unlimited logical power of networks of neuron-like elements.

It is debated now whether cybernetics has lived up to its early promises, and whether we can expect further advances in our understanding of the brain from this approach. The same can be said about pushing further the analogy between brains and computers.

There are parallels, of course, and they afford us some insight into brain mechanisms. In both cases we can speak of a network of elementary units—neurons in one and transistors in the other. The all-or-none action potentials make the neurons somewhat analogous to bistable units in electronics, which are the building blocks of the binary logic used by computers: a unit is *on* or *off;* a statement is *true* or *false;* and in a *computer,* a cipher is 0 or 1.

But real neurons are far more complex. Not only can they have thousands of inputs but the strengths of the signals necessary to trigger them, the *thresholds*, depend on many other changeable factors. McCulloch, in his study of the logical properties in networks of neurons, coined the expression "impoverished neuron" to denote a hypothetical neuron that is deprived of many of its biological properties and acts more like a simple electronic switch. This clearly makes it easier to calculate what would happen in a complicated network of such elements. Of course, one worries about the function of the features that were neglected.

Nevertheless, whatever else goes on in the brain, neurons are engaged in some form of *logical calculus*. A primitive example of such an action is shown in Fig. 2.13. Here neurons 1, 2, and 3 are "impoverished neurons." Neuron 1 is triggered by an event called A, neuron 2 by an event called B. Neuron 1 makes an excitatory synapse (arrow) on neuron 3. The firing of neuron 3 is called event C. Neuron 2 also makes a synapse with neuron 3, but the connection is inhibitory (dot). The firing of neuron 2 will prevent neuron 3 from firing. The logical

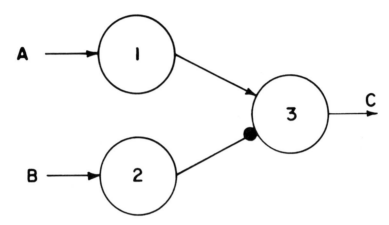

2.13 *A logical network of neurons*

function of this circuit is thus: Event C will occur if A has occurred, providing B has *not* occurred. Logicians sometimes express such a function by a *truth table* such as the following:

If A is:	and B is:	then C is:
NO	NO	NO
YES	NO	YES
NO	YES	NO
YES	YES	NO

This gives the status C for the four combinations of binary choices for A and B. Thus we read from left to right: If there is no A and no B, then there will be no C; if there is A but no B, then there will be C, etc.

Networks of many such neuron-like units were studied by the Italian physicist and cybernetician, Eduardo Caianiello. The late Frank Rosenblatt of Cornell University designed a system composed of impoverished neurons that was capable of learning simple discrimination tasks. He called it the *perceptron*. In our own laboratory at Syracuse University, we have used large computers to study the dynamics of neural networks containing up to thousands of neuron-like elements. This is still a small number compared with the vast populations of neurons that communicate with one another in the human brain. One of our earlier studies, in which we tried to construct a model of associative memory, is described in Chapter 3.

The difficulty with all such efforts is, of course, that the details of the connections between neurons in the real brain are not known, and if they were known, their complexity would make it all but impossible to calculate what might happen in such a system. The only real model of a brain, it has been pointed out, is another brain.

Receptors, effectors, and reflexes

Let us return now to live neurons. To complete our very sketchy picture of the organization of the brain, we must say something about the neurons at the periphery of the nervous system, the *receptors* and the *effectors*.

A *receptor* is an element which in engineering language would be called a *transducer*. It has the characteristics of translating one physical variable into another. A pressure gauge is a transducer; it changes pressure into the movement of a pointer along a scale. Similarly, the rod and cone cells of the eye are sensitive to light impinging on the retina and respond with electric signals. These signals are then passed on from neuron to neuron in the manner previously described. In the same way, other senses have their specialized receptors: the touch receptors in the skin, the chemoreceptors of smell and taste, and so forth. In the case of vision, the electric signals from the rod and cone cells are transmitted to a variety of neurons in the retina. The last layer of these is formed by the so-called *retinal ganglion cells* whose axons—about a million of them all bundled together—form the optic nerve. (We now understand the nature of a nerve: It is a bundle of axons carrying signals from one part of the nervous system to another.)

Of the *effectors* we will mention only one type, the *motoneuron*. It sends its axon to a muscle fiber, where a synapse produces postsynaptic potentials which cause the muscle to contract. Look again at the grand scheme of the nervous system in Fig. 2.8. Our brain now appears simply as a link between receptors and effectors, a grandiose elaboration of the most primitive neural system: the *reflex arc*.

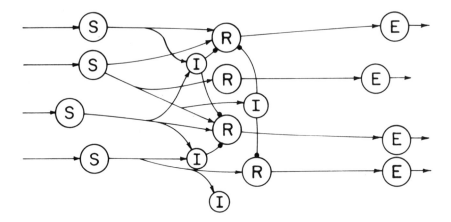

2.14 *Neural circuit diagram for a simple reflex. Sense receptors, S, are connected to effectors E, through a group of relay neurons, R, and interneurons, I.*

In some of the lowest multicellular animals, the nervous system is not much more than a few receptor cells, a few effector cells, and a few neurons in between. These are the *relay neurons* and *interneurons* (Fig. 2.14), and in higher forms they will evolve into a brain. But even in man such primitive systems have survived and form an important part of our nervous system. Our simplest reflexes do not even have relay neurons and interneurons. In these *monosynaptic* reflexes, the afferent, sensory fibers synapse directly on the motoneurons. Motor response is involuntary and simply determined by the stimulus. The patellar reflex, or knee jerk, is probably the best-known example of this.

Feature detectors

A simple scheme like the one described above would be inadequate for most tasks of everyday life. Fine distinctions have to be made between different stimuli, and the response generally requires the activation of many muscles, often with precise timing among them. The hare must instantly distinguish between a fox and another hare and behave accordingly. Such tasks require, on the input side, neural structures that can recognize patterns, and, on the output side, the storage of programs of action that can be released upon a simple command. For example, the eye of the frog has special detectors for small moving shapes. Triggering these *"bug detectors"* releases a fixed behavioral pattern—the turning toward and striking at the bug. The term *tropism* is sometimes used to denote such genetically determined motor programs. The neural circuits that generate these automatic types of behavior are called *feature generators*. The swallowing reflex in man may be an automatic response to certain stimuli, or the result of voluntary action. In either case it involves many muscles, activated in a preprogrammed sequence over which we have relatively little control once the sequence is initiated.

In some invertebrates there exist single neurons that release more or less complex programs of action. Such *command neurons* presumably trigger a feature-generating network. It is reasonable to suppose that the command neurons in turn are activated by feature detectors. The chain of events making up this type of reflex is as follows: Signals from a particular sense organ are analyzed by a feature detector. If the presence of the feature in question is established, a feature generator is triggered, sometimes via a single command neuron. The feature generator releases a predetermined action program that is the response appropriate to the detected feature. There are numerous examples of such reflex chains in primitive animals and in man. We know about these from behavioral studies, but only in a few cases do we know all the neural circuits that go with them.

One of the most significant advances in recent years has been a discovery by David Hubel and Torsten Wiesel of Harvard University Medical School that some neurons in the neocortex of mammals appear to be detectors of special features in the world we see. Hubel and Wiesel have classified these cells as *simple, complex,* and *hypercomplex*. Although the patterns to which they respond are rather primitive —lines, bars, edges of different locations and orientations in the visual field—some physiologists believe they are the elements from which more complicated patterns are built up at higher centers. In this view each recognizable visual pattern is represented somewhere in the brain by a single neuron. One of these, for example, would be involved in the recognition of a particular face, say your grandmother's. Somewhat facetiously, such hypothetical cells have been called *grandmother neurons*.

The neocortex:
a view of the summit

Let us now return to the question of structure in the nervous system of man.

The human brain represents the end result, at least for the time being, of the enormous development of the uppermost part of the vertebrate nervous system. This steady shift to the top is called *encephalization.* From the upper portion of the spinal cord, three structures have evolved. Starting from the top, they are the *forebrain,* the *midbrain,* and the *hindbrain.* These structures are recognizable in all vertebrates. In the higher mammals a new structure appears: the *neocortex,* or the *cerebral cortex.* It gains in size and importance as we go up the evolutionary ladder. In man it makes up about 83 percent of the total brain weight and nearly covers all the older brain structures. Its deeply convoluted surface, shown so graphically in Vesalius's engraving (Fig. 2.6, page 44), represents structurally and functionally the very *top* of the human nervous system. We like to believe that our massive neocortex is responsible for all the so-called *higher functions* and all the subtle differences that distinguish man from his nearest intellectual competitor in the animal kingdom. It has been called our *thinking cap.*

We have thus assigned an up-down direction to the human nervous system: *up* is toward the neocortex, *down* is away from the neocortex and toward the older, *lower* structures in the brain. All these structures are interconnected by information-carrying cables made up of axons. Following the up-down concept, we speak of *ascending* and *descending* pathways, and, as in the case of the afferent and efferent nerves linking the brain with the periphery, the ascending pathways can be described as carrying information *toward* the neocortex, and descending pathways as relaying commands to the lower structures.

As we shall see, this picture of a strict hierarchy in the brain is an oversimplification and has been the source of many misconceptions. It is nevertheless a start, and we can carry it a little further when we look more closely at the neocortex itself.

Imagine a sheet measuring about two and a half square feet and a little less than one eighth of an inch thick, made up of over ten billion neurons. Add on one side of this sheet a thick layer of fibers, the axons coming into and going out of this structure, and we have a rudimentary picture of the neocortex. To complete the picture we must do two things: divide the sheet into two halves for the two distinct brain hemispheres, and crumple these structures to fit into our braincase (look again at Fig. 2.6). The two halves communicate with each other through a thick band of axons, the *corpus callosum,* seen in the cleft between the two brain halves in Fig. 2.6. Through this connection, information received by either brain half is shared with the other. In Fig. 2.15 I have tried to show a very much simplified conception of the

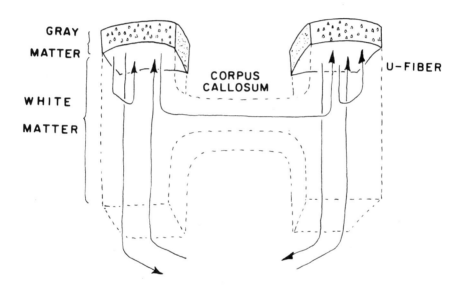

2.15 *Architecture of the neocortex showing two patches of neocortex, one from each brain half. Fibers are shown entering and leaving the* gray *matter from below: U-fibers going from one neuron to another in the same brain half;* callosal *fibers going from one brain half to the other; and the fibers entering and leaving the cortex.*

structure of the neocortex: the two thin sheets of neurons, also called *gray matter,* and below them the axon fibers, or *white matter.* Some of these axons go from one brain half to the other (via the *corpus callosum*). Some go from one part of the neocortex to another part on the same side; these are called U-fibers. The rest go to or come from lower brain structures.

What distinguishes the neocortex from other parts of the brain is its striking uniformity. Apart from a crumpled appearance, it shows to the naked eye about as much structure as smooth peanut butter spread on a piece of toast. Even under the miscroscope the structure of the individual neurons and the interconnections between them are remarkably uniform over the entire cortical area. This is especially true for those portions of the cortex called the *sensory cortex* that receive the incoming sensory signals of touch, hearing, and sight. Figure 2.16

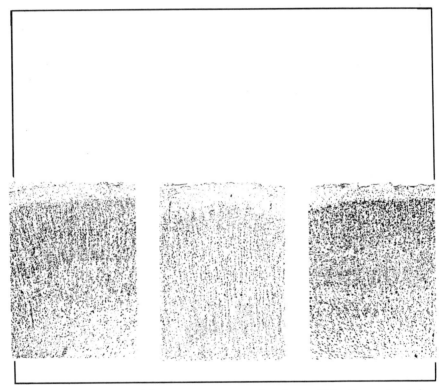

2.16 *Three sections of human neocortex showing cell bodies only, taken from areas that receive the sensory information of touch, hearing, and vision. (From* The Isocortex of Man, *P. Bailey and G. von Bonin, University of Illinois Press, 1951)*

shows the distribution of cell bodies in three widely different portions of the neocortex. The thin layer of gray matter shown schematically in Fig. 2.15 is greatly enlarged. The three sections are from different sensory areas. Apart from slightly different thicknesses and cell sizes, the three look very much the same. This feature is responsible for the name *isocortex*, meaning *equal* cortex, which is often used instead of *neocortex*. (By now it should be obvious that neuroanatomists are fond of inventing new names.)

To appreciate the meaning of a picture like Fig. 2.16, it must be pointed out that only cell bodies are shown here. In addition, each neuron has an extensive tree of dendrites and an axon that branches repeatedly within the gray matter and sends one branch out into the white matter. Fig. 2.17 shows a few selected neurons in the neocortex

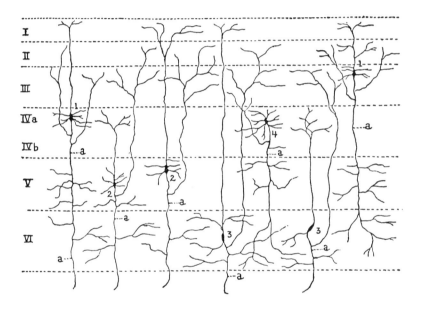

2.17 *Different cell types in the neocortex. Axons are labelled a. All other fibers are dendrites. The gray matter here is divided into six main layers. White matter is below layer VI. (From* Human Neuroanatomy, *M. B. Carpenter, 7th ed., Williams & Wilkins, Baltimore, Md., 1976)*

with their typical fiber trees. Put together Figs. 2.15, 2.16, and 2.17 and visualize every cubic millimeter (the size of a pin head) of neocortex containing between thirty and one hundred thousand neurons, criss-crossed by about a mile of axons, and you may get a feeling of the incredible delicacy and high density of cortical structure.

But does this cortical maze represent structure, or randomness, or a combination of the two? And if the latter, what fractions can we ascribe to either one? Is the isocortex, which superficially looks the same all over, precisely wired in every microscopic detail, or is it more nearly like the "bowlful of porridge" which is its gross appearance?

These questions are important and will be discussed in greater detail in Chapter 3. In the meantime, we face a perplexing problem. Here, where the functions are most diverse and sophisticated, we are looking at the monotonously uniform goo of gray matter. And we are also reminded of the other puzzle mentioned before: the combination of structural delicacy and functional ruggedness.

The functions generally attributed to the neocortex include detection of features in all sensory systems; learning and association of new features and learning of all kinds; memory and recall of sequences of events perceived in the past; patterning of elaborate programs of voluntary muscle actions from tying shoelaces to playing Liszt; formation and understanding of speech; creativity and appreciation in all forms of art, and of course all sensations and consciousness.

A closer look at the axons emerging from the bottom of the neocortex is instructive. Look again at Fig. 2.15. All in all there are about ten billion fibers over the entire two and one half square feet of neocortical area. Two hundred million of them cross from one hemisphere to the other, forming the *corpus callosum*. But the majority of the axons dip down into the white matter, only to reemerge and enter the cortex at a different point. These are the so-called U-fibers. Only about one in a thousand of the fibers entering the cortex at any point is an axon that comes from lower structures and brings in sensory information. All others are either U-fibers or *callosal* fibers and thus represent *cortex talking to cortex*. This remarkable fact was pointed out by Valentino Braitenberg[6], and we will refer to it again later. It points to the highly *reflective* mode of operation of the neocortex. If we were to compare it to a government, it would be analogous to a group of people in lively dispute with one another, but virtually isolated from the outside world. However, unlike this caricature of a *bad* government, the cortex *knows* what is going on outside, most of the time even before it happens! The picture now flashing onto my retina is mostly obsolete by the time the information reaches the neocortex because the cortex has already *computed ahead* on the basis of previous information. When a scene of nature is observed, such as the one described on page 19, the neocortex *knows* that some of the elements are permanent and others transitory. The mountain will not have moved, but a falling leaf will be predictably closer and closer to the ground in successive instances. The new images thus serve mostly to confirm what is already known and to make small corrections. Meanwhile, the neocortex is *reminded* by the falling leaf of the coming of autumn, and from that reminder may be led to other thoughts.

Although the structural aspects of the neocortex are nearly uniform throughout, we can distinguish a number of areas whose functions are reasonably well defined. Again, the overall plan is repeated here. Some regions receive sensory information that is relayed from subcortical regions; others issue orders to muscles. Still others do neither. We are not really sure what they do.

If you look back at Fig. 2.8, you think of the neocortex as making up the tip of the pyramid. Like the lower structures, it has well-defined input and output regions. As an example, the visual information comes in via a relay station in the forebrain, the *thalamus*, at a place in the neocortex called the *visual projection area*. We will describe these pathways in more detail in the next chapter.

Jumping once again to the motor end of the neocortex, we find regions from which the voluntary muscles are controlled, all neatly laid out like a map of the body itself. But the bulk of the human cortex still lies beyond these regions, with all the functions cited above still unaccounted for. A few regions adjoining sensory and motor areas have been explored by physiologists. There are *association areas* where sensory inputs from different senses are mixed. There are islands here and there where something is known about function, such as the areas responsible for speech. It should be made quite clear however that we are far from having any plausible neural mechanism that could account for human speech. Of the speech area in the neocortex we know only that any damage to it will result in speech impairment. Structurally, the neocortex looks not much different there than anywhere else.

The puzzle of structural monotony and functional diversity was addressed by O.D. Creutzfeldt[7]. He believed that what makes a particular part of the cortex specialize in processing visual information or handle olfactory or tactile inputs has little to do with intrinsic structural differences in these parts. "Specific functions," according to Creutzfeldt, "are defined by the origin of its afferents and the destination of its efferent connections." He sees the cortex only as "a link in the stream of activities from the thalamus and other afferent structures to the effectors."

Our intuition tells us that as we go away from the projection areas, we are going toward *higher* brain centers, perhaps toward higher and more complex intellectual functions, and that as we approach the motor output areas, we are descending again toward more peripheral areas. This reasoning might lead us to conclude that somewhere in the vast unexplored region in between there must be a *pinnacle*, an absolute center, the ultimate destiny of all incoming information and the absolute authority over all issuing commands. Sherrington some time ago conjectured that perhaps a single neuron somewhere in the neocortex had that distinction. He called it the *pontifical neuron*. He apparently soon discarded this notion in favor of a more democratic system in which decisions were made by *populations* of neurons.

But the concept of a cerebral center or summit lingers on stubbornly, in spite of the fact that neither structure nor function offers any evidence of its existence. A somewhat milder form of this scheme is proposed by some neurophysiologists, who believe there are many single neuron centers throughout the neocortex, including the feature-detecting *grandmother* neurons. Following the ecclesiastical nomenclature stated by Sherrington, these are sometimes called *cardinals*, and some undoubtedly exist. We have already encountered the *command* neurons in invertebrate nervous systems. There is also one report—but only one and it is several years old—of a neuron in the neocortex of a monkey that was found to respond selectively when the monkey was shown the image of a hand.[8] What is perhaps more significant is the fact that, with the single exception of the monkey hand detector, no single neurons have been found that are detectors for features more complex than bars and edges of light, despite very concentrated searches in many laboratories.

3

HANG-UPS IN NEUROSCIENCE

Gewöhnlich glaubt der Mensch, wenn er nur Worte hört,
Es müsse sich dabei doch auch was denken lassen.

(When they hear words, most people think
There must be something worth pondering.)
—GOETHE, Faust, I

Just as wars are invariably between *two* sides, so controversies in science tend to harden into dichotomies. In physics the question of the nature of light took on this duel aspect when Newton postulated that it consisted of a stream of particles and Christian Huygens believed it to be a wave. This situation remained until the twentieth century when De Broglie and Bohr and Heisenberg showed that both theories were valid aspects, and the particle-wave controversy turned into the particle-wave duality.

In neuroscience several pairs of such opposing viewpoints have emerged and attracted some passionate advocates. Yet no clear resolution of any of these conflicts has emerged, as it has in the case of the particle-wave controversy. Meanwhile, the unresolved issues have assumed a significance greater than their due and have tended to color the opinions on many related questions. For this reason I have called them *hang-ups*. They distract and cause *syndromes* of opinions. My intention in discussing them is not so much to express an opinion one way or another as perhaps to lay to rest some issues that have become more emotional than substantive. I will show also that, just as in the case of the particle-wave duality in physics, alternative solutions which appeared as incompatible opposites may in some unexpected ways turn out to be integrated in an eventual solution.

Atomism and globalism

The theory according to which single neurons, *cardinals* if you will, represent complex perceptual features or abstract concepts is sometimes called *atomism* in neuroscience. The term is of course metaphoric and probably cannot be defined too rigidly. It suggests, on the one hand, that the elementary unit of neuronal structure, the *neuron,* is also an elementary *cognitive* unit. It is also taken to mean that the concepts themselves are built up in the fashion of complex molecules from a set of elementary building blocks, or *atoms.* In the case of visual concepts, these elementary parts are perhaps the simple linear patterns for which Hubel and Wiesel have found detectors in the neocortex. Such a viewpoint tends to favor a highly deterministic outlook in which the processing proceeds from sensory input to cognitive unit by a rigid *pulse logic* similar to a computer's.

In this scheme the brain appears to be an elaboration of a simple mechanism in the nervous system of the marine worm, *Myxicola infundibulum,* described by M.B.V. Roberts.[1] This animal buries itself in the sand near the water's edge. A small crown of tentacles normally protrudes above the surface of the sand to feed on small bits of organic matter and to draw oxygen from the water. Its nervous system has a prominent neuron which triggers *one* action, making what is probably the only decision of which this primitive creature is capable: to withdraw rapidly into the sand at any sign of danger. Such a task requires a nervous system that is equipped with a *feature detector*, which can distinguish between *danger* and *no danger,* and a *feature generator,* which stores the action program. Linking the two is the single *command neuron.* Figure 3.1 illustrates how the feature detector will trigger the command neuron, which in turn triggers the feature generator. The nervous system thus carries out the logical function "if danger, then withdraw."

Physiologists tend to favor such atomistic schemes because there is an intuitive simplicity about the concepts. In the case of the human

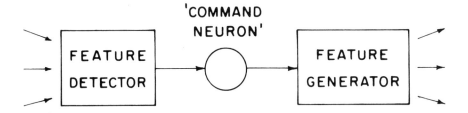

3.1 *Example of a reflex involving feature detection and feature generation. A command neuron is triggered when a particular feature is contained in the sensory input, and it then releases a specific motor program.*

brain, one is tempted to think that all the sifted, analyzed sensory information or the results of all thought processes reach their final expression in the firing of certain neurons that have special significance attached to them, almost like labels attached to indicator lights on a control panel. Thus at the highest stage of neural processing, the state of the outside world could be read off by some *operator* with a glance at the bank of cardinal neurons. Indeed, so close is the apparent analogy that the metaphor is used both ways: The nerve center is thought of as a *control room,* and real control rooms are called *nerve centers.*

There is another reason for the relative popularity of this view. The 1940's saw the rapid development of an experimental technique that enabled neurophysiologists to *tune in* and record the activity of single neurons of experimental animals. The method consists of inserting minute electrodes into nervous tissue. These *microelectrodes* are either very thin pointed wires of tungsten coated with lacquer so that only the very tip makes electrical contact, or glass pipettes drawn out to a very fine tip and filled with a conducting liquid. The electrode tips can be placed either very close to a neuron or actually within a neuron cell body. The electrical signals picked up in this way are then amplified and can be displayed on an oscilloscope or recorded on tape. When heard through a loudspeaker, each action potential produces a sharp click, and an active neuron emits a lively sustained crackling sound.

With the development of the microelectrode technique, much of neurophysiology became a study of individual neurons. It is possible, for instance, to listen to a single neuron in the neocortex of a cat or monkey while the animal is presented with different visual or auditory stimuli. One can then attempt to relate these responses to the types of stimuli presented. If a neuron is found to respond in an especially lively and consistent fashion to a particular stimulus, it is said to be a *detector* of that stimulus. This term implies that the characteristic response of this neuron is actually *used* by the nervous system to detect the feature with which the experimenter has found it to be associated. It thus attaches *meaning* to the activity of individual neurons. This, of course, *is* the atomistic viewpoint.

There are a number of difficulties with this interpretation. We are once again confronted with the control-room metaphor, which is beginning to wear thin. Why should individual neurons be indicators of this or that feature? Are we to believe that there is an analogy to the operator who sits in front of the control panel and scans the lights? And if we reject the idea of a nonphysical homunculus ensconced in our neocortex, then why feature detectors? The currently popular *psycho-neural identity theory* asserts that the firing of certain neurons simply *is* the perception of the smell of a rose or of a skunk.

But here we run into another difficulty. A neuron is a living cell covered over its entire body, including all its projecting fibers, with a continuous wall, the cell membrane. It is a tiny island living in a sea of extracellular fluid. Its only communication with other neurons is through the chemical messengers that occasionally stream across the narrow gaps separating it from other cells. When the molecules impinge on the cell membrane, they cause the small voltage fluctuations we described, and if these fluctuations are in the right direction and sufficiently strong, the cell will fire. Again, its own firing is an event known to the world outside its boundaries only by virtue of the streams of molecules *it* secretes into the intercellular spaces. But can we say that the neuron *knows* the signals it received are traceable to an olfactory sense that has picked up the smell of a rose? Horace Barlow[2] actually suggests that "a central neuron is reaching out to discover something important about what is happening in the real objective world." But it seems difficult to attribute curiosity and knowledge to a single cell buried somewhere in our neocortex. While we cannot rule out the possibility that single neurons are *sentient atoms* in our system, it does not seem like a very plausible idea. But if the neuron that detects a feature doesn't *know* it, then who or what does?

We are drawn here into what Gilbert Ryle has called a "category mistake." When we talk about a neuron, we talk about electrochemical processes occurring on its cell membrane, and when we talk about perception, we talk about our *sensation* of *what is out there*. These are different *categories*, according to Ryle. We should talk about one *or* the other, but not mix them. However, the atomistic view in its strictest sense is an assertion that there is no category barrier between the two. Quoting again from Barlow's paper, "Single Units and Sensation," we are told that "we should not use phrases like 'unit activity reflects, reveals, or monitors thought processes' because the activities of neurons quite simply *are* thought processes."

An alternative set of viewpoints, in which meaning resides in the activity of large numbers or *populations* of neurons, is sometimes called *globalism*. The opposing concepts of atomism and globalism as used here are somewhat analogous to, but not identical with, what Steven Rose[3] and others have called *reductionism and holism,* or to George Somjen's pair of concepts, *localization* and *equipotentiality.*[4] This only shows that the many possible opinions are readily sorted into different pairs of opposing viewpoints.

I will use the term *globalism* simply to denote the belief that single neurons in the human brain are rarely the carriers of complex information. They merely *participate*, along with many other cells, in registering a perception, expressing a thought, making a decision, or issuing a command. Globalists, like Walter J. Freeman of Berkeley, talk of *cooperative activities* in *neural masses*, and of waves of activity spreading through populations of neurons.

When a physiologist monitors a single neuron with his microelectrode, he should, in the globalist's view, not search for complex meanings. The activity he records is at best a very weak representation of what really counts: the combined activity of thousands, perhaps millions of neurons. The word *gestalt* suggests itself here. If cognition resides in the activity of a population of neurons, then it may be surmised that characteristic *patterns* of such activity carry specific meanings. Implicit in the idea of *gestalt* is a certain variability, which in turn suggests that we may allow a certain amount of noise or randomness or even error to creep into the neural mechanism without seriously affecting its proper functioning.

This touches on another controversy in neuroscience, which we will soon discuss, that between determinism and randomness. Globalist models, as we have seen, allow a looseness in both structure and function, and hence make possible the assumption of randomness. Note that this does not mean there is a necessary connection between the two views but, rather, a frequent concurrence, a *syndrome*, to use a medical expression. Similarly, atomism, pulse logic, and strict determinism tend to run together. With or without randomness, global models also suggest a certain *redundancy*. After all, many neurons are invoked here to account for something that atomists believe can be done by one.

Globalism has in general been less popular with neurophysiologists than its rival, atomism. One of the objections has been that globalist theories are not readily tested by present experimental techniques. A single microelectrode placed inside a cell body will record the activity of this cell only. *Extracellular* microelectrodes may pick up signals from a small cluster of neurons. Techniques have now been developed for recording with multiple electrodes the simultaneous chatter of ten or more neurons in different brain locations. Such advanced recording techniques are not only technically difficult but they present the experimenter with massive data that can only be described as overwhelming. Having obtained the data, it is not at all clear what to do with them. The physiologist's task here is a peculiar one. He intercepts a message somewhere in the neocortex and—by looking at oscilloscopes or reading graphs or listening to tapes—presents this message to the very periphery of his own nervous system. But the code is inappropriate for that stage, and the message makes no sense. What we are trying to do can be likened to sampling a spoonful of liver bile and trying to figure out from its taste, what it does in our intestines. There also remains the very fundamental question of whether or not we have even captured a substantial portion of the central message.

A more modest and in some ways a more fruitful experimental approach to neural mass action is to measure gross properties of nerve tissue rather than individual action potentials. This can be done by attaching electrodes to various points on the outside of the human skull. The resulting traces of what is called the electroencephalogram (EEG) have been studied extensively ever since they were discovered by Hans Berger in the late 1920's. But the information contained in the squiggly lines of the EEG is limited. Some gross pathologies can be detected, and some very gross categories of mental stages (attention, drowsiness, sleep) show distinct and recognizable EEG patterns. The encephalographer has been compared to a geologist who uses the records from a seismograph to infer events deep within the earth. Actually the comparison is an understatement. The geologist has a fair understanding of the propagation of seismic waves and their relation to shifting masses below the earth's surface. Such a basic understanding is still lacking in the case of the EEG.

There is another, more profound difficulty with the globalist postulate that mass action, or perhaps the simultaneous activities in a *constellation* of neurons, carries meaning. Again it has to do with the concept of attaching a *label* to neural activity, but this time the label goes with a population of neurons, not a single neuron. And again we tend to look for a *ghost* that observes this activity to get us out of the category of blinking neurons and into the category of thought. Barring that, we must somehow explain why this particular group of quite ordinary neurons has a *collective knowledge* of the smell of a rose wafting beneath my nose.

In recent years a technique has become popular in which many EEG traces are superimposed according to the timing of an external stimulus. The averaging techniques used include some rather sophisticated electronics to extract reproducible features out of the irregular and rather unpredictable EEG traces. The so-called *evoked potentials* which emerge tell us much about when and how our nervous systems reacts to external stimuli. We will discuss some of these findings in Chapter 5.

Very recently some new techniques have been developed which provide scientists with an entirely new vista of the living brain. It was observed that blood flow to different parts of the nervous system is delicately controlled by the vascular system. Neural activity consumes energy just as muscular activity does. An active brain part demands more oxygen, and more blood must be rushed to the site. Thus if we could map the flow of blood through the brain when it carries out a particular task, we would "see" what parts are busy at the time.

Scientists at the University of Lund in Sweden have succeeded in doing just that.[5] The method consists of introducing a radioactive substance into a patient's bloodstream and observing the gamma rays coming from the brain. A map of the brain surface can be constructed in which different areas show varying degrees of activity. In the resting, inattentive brain, most of the activity is found in the so-called prefrontal cortex. This area is believed to reflect the' brain's *inner thoughts,* that is, its preoccupation with past events and planning for the future. When attention is directed to sensory stimuli, or when action is called for by the brain, the pattern of activity is quite different. In Fig.3.2 we see the "activity portrait" of the brain in its inattentive state (a), and when the subject is speaking (b). In the second case we see three distinct brain areas activated: the *supplementary motor area* (1), which is concerned with the programming of sequential actions; the motor and sensory areas directly involved in speech production—

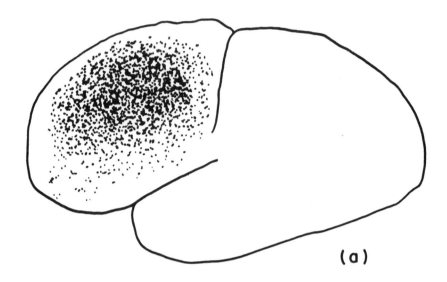

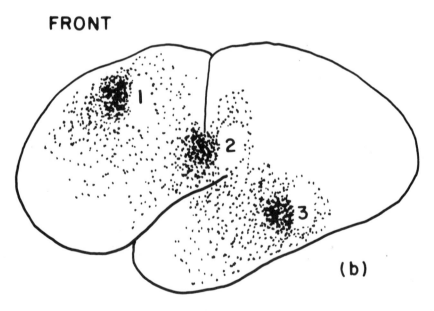

3.2 *Brain portraits from a study of blood flow. Areas showing a high radioactivity are shaded. (Redrawn from "Brain Function and Blood Flow," N. A. Lassen, D. H. Ingvar, and E. Skinhøj, Scientific American 239:62, 1978)*

the mouth, tongue, and larynx—(2); and the auditory area of the cortex (3).

Increased energy consumption in active brain centers can be followed also by putting a radioactive tag on glucose, the fuel used by neurons. For this purpose a slightly altered molecule called *2-deoxyglucose* is used. It is taken up by the energy-hungry cells and accumulates there, since it cannot be metabolized. A particularly powerful method called *positron emission tomography* (PET) uses radioactive labels that emit positive electrons, or *positrons*. This allows the experimenter to observe patterns of neural activity in selected cross sections of the living brain.

The blood-flow studies and positron emission tomography have enormous potential. Unlike the techniques of microelectrode recording, they are *noninvasive*; they require no opening of the skull, no piercing of the brain tissue. It may be expected that just as the introduction of microelectrode techniques in the forties caused neuroscientists to emphasize the role of single neurons, so these new techniques will cause interest to shift toward larger brain centers and the functioning of larger populations of cells.

Determinism and randomness

"The nervous system is not a random net. Its units are not redundant. Its organization is highly specific, not merely in terms of the connections between particular neurons, but also in terms of the number, style, and location of terminals upon different parts of the same cell and the precise distribution of terminals arising from that cell.[6]

This often-quoted statement by Sanford Palay, a Harvard University neuroanatomist, marks an extreme position. Let us see what is at issue here.

The characteristic structural features of every human are determined by an inherited blueprint contained in the molecules of DNA (deoxyribonucleic acid), in which the features, both actual and latent, from our two parents are combined. Characteristics known to be determined in this way lie at both ends of the scale of structures that constitute our bodies. They include the gross features of physical stature and body type, color of hair and eyes; and perhaps also such mental and emotional features as ambition, a tendency toward artistic expression, and others. At the other end of the scale, we know that precise structures of large molecules are likewise specified by the parental determinants: the nucleic acids, DNA among them, which are themselves the carriers of genetic information, and the proteins. Among the latter group are the *histocompatibility antigens*, proteins which are our most personal possession, since they define for each of us a uniqueness, or *selfhood*. They are recognized as our own by the immune system that throughout our lifetime guards us against incursions by alien structures. The selfhood of the proteins is entirely genetic; it is a thing apart from that other selfhood which is largely experiential and is expressed in our central nervous system.

The range and the limitations of genetic determinacy can be examined by studying identical twins, whose genetic blueprints are known to be identical. We are all familiar with twins' startling similarity of physical appearance. On the other hand, it is known that the lives of twins often take strikingly dissimilar turns. This may be due in part to different environmental influences, but perhaps also to some native differences which are however not genetic. We know, for example, that the physical similarity does not include fine structural details. Their noses may look identical, but the pattern of pores would be different when examined under a magnifying glass. Their hands may have identical *features*, but the precise pattern of veins will be different, and so, I am told, would be their fingerprints.

It appears that the genetic blueprint specifies mostly characteristics at the two ends of the structural scale, allowing details in the intermediate range to be filled in by chance. In a given piece of tissue, made up of a large number of cells of certain sizes and shapes, the exact position of each cell may be irrelevant to the functioning of that tissue. A viable organism would develop even though these details were unspecified by the DNA molecules. But how are the unspecified characteristics *filled in*? We said *by chance,* but what does this really mean?

Physicists have pondered such questions in connection with macroscopic physical systems. They attribute to *chance* any process whose detailed mechanisms are hidden for one reason or another. The throw of dice is a matter of *chance*, since the outcome depends on the precise way the dice tumble through the air, and on the roughness, elasticity, and minute details of the surface they strike before coming to rest. In this case the factors determining the outcome are too numerous and too minute to be controlled or foreseen. We can conceive of a mechanical dice thrower made so precisely that a seven, or any other combination, can be thrown with certainty, simply by setting some controls on the machine. In practice, it is unlikely that the condition of the surfaces and the initial motion of the dice can be held to a precision that insures a certain outcome. An absolute limit to this precision is given by the uncontrollable "thermal" motions of dice, table, and the intervening air. Similarly, the exact path followed by a bolt of lightning may depend on processes occurring on a molecular scale, such as minute fluctuations in the density of air ions along the path. We will say more in Chapter 6 about the indeterminacy of processes which depend on the random motions that are always present on the scale of atoms and molecules. Such microscopic fluctuations are frequently *amplified*, as in the case of lightning. The *microcosm* is thus a steady reservoir of unpredictability, feeding large fluctuations into the macrocosm by way of minute effects acting upon critically poised processes.

The agents of what we have called *chance* are thus processes affecting the outcome of a macroscopic event in unpredictable ways, either because they are too numerous to be determined with sufficient accuracy or because they depend on random molecular motions and are therefore *fundamentally* unknowable. Without specifying the processes further, we will refer to them collectively as the *accidents of nature*. The path of lightning is governed by such accidents. So is the pattern of waves on the surface of a body of water. We can predict the *average* size of a wave if we know the winds, temperatures, and depth of the water. But *when* and *where* a wave of a given size will appear depends again on the accidents of nature. Gross features are generally predictable, details are not.

Let us return now to the question raised above, which was how the structure of a piece of tissue can be *filled in* when only the molecules and some parameters of gross structure are predetermined. The answer is again that these features are given by the accidents of nature—by chance. Undoubtedly the microstructure of most organs is determined this way. It is clear that an organ such as the heart is relatively insensitive to very small variations in structure. As long as an unbroken wall separates the two ventricles, as long as the valves fit reasonably well, and as long as the muscle is assured of an adequate blood supply, the heart will give us little trouble.

In the brain, by contrast, it may be of vital importance that a particular group of neurons makes synaptic contact with a particular other neuron. But this would mean that, unlike in the design of other organs, the small details of brain structure cannot be left to chance. Is it possible then that the brain's microstructure is predetermined in every detail? This is the contention of structural determinists like Palay. Can such a detailed blueprint be contained in the DNA molecule? Let us see how much information would be required for this.

Assume that there are exactly ten billion neurons in the brain, and that each neuron makes a thousand synaptic contacts with other neurons. There are thus a thousand times ten billion, or ten trillion, synapses whose locations must be specified. The ways in which such information may be expressed, or *encoded*, are studied in a branch of science called *information theory*. We will not concern ourselves here with this subject, but merely point out that the encoding can be done, for example, by using a string of numbers, or the letters of the English alphabet, or the molecular language of DNA. Suppose we were to print out this information in some form, indicating for each synapse the cell of origin and the cell of destination. If we printed 5000 letters to a page and 500 pages to a volume, we would require about 100 million such volumes! It is impossible that this much information is genetically determined. In fact, it exceeds the total capacity of human DNA by almost a millionfold.

Does this prove then that most of the delicate neural circuitry in our brain is left to chance? Not quite. It would still be possible to have strict structural determinism, even with our limited genetic information, if we included certain rules of *order* and *symmetry*. For example, in an amorphous substance such as glass, the molecules occupy more or less random positions in the solid. If we were to tell someone the precise location of every molecule in even a small chunk of glass (assuming this could be done), an enormous amount of information would be required. The situation is shown in Fig. 3.3 by a hundred dots scattered at random, in which every dot represents a molecule in the solid body. On the other hand, if the same molecules formed an orderly array, as they do in a crystal, it would suffice to give just a few numbers to locate every molecule with great precision. In the case of the "crystal" shown in Fig. 3.3 (b), we can describe the entire structure simply as "a ten-by-ten-square lattice with one quarter-inch between points."

Similarly, in the case of the brain the specifications needed could be greatly reduced if some general rules of symmetry were to apply. The fact that neurons, such as the ones shown in Figs. 2.9 or 2.17 (pages 50 and 65), have *typical* structures means that there are such rules.

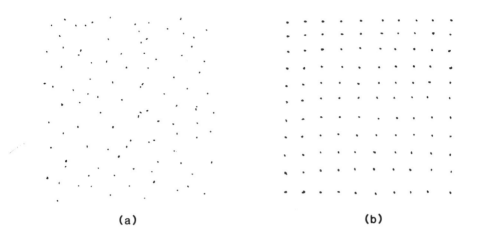

(a)   (b)

3.3 (a) *Amorphous solid. Molecules are distributed at random.* **(b)** *Two-dimensional diagram of a crystal lattice. Molecules form a very regular array.*

The question remains whether the acquired information can be sufficiently reduced in this way, and whether all the remaining information is determined by our genes.

A frequent argument against any *looseness* in the design is the statement that there is "mounting evidence" for structural determinism. This means that new rules and similarities between brains are continually being discovered. But this is not surprising, since practically all neuroanatomical research is a search for such regularities. Any *result* therefore is additional evidence for structure, but the absence of results may merely mean that we have not looked hard enough, or that we have not looked in the right places. Randomness, by its very nature, is much harder to demonstrate than determinism. Unlike the sequence of atoms in most manmade polymers or chain molecules, the sequence of nucleotides in a molecule of DNA *appears* to be random, but of course it is not.

There is, incidentally, a common confusion about the concept of *randomness*. The term does not imply that everything is random, but merely that *some* features of the structure are left to chance. Some of the negative reactions among anatomists to any suggestion of randomness can be attributed to this misunderstanding, and also to early attempts by *brain theorists* to disregard much of the known structure and regularities and to talk about *self-organizing systems*, as though a functioning brain could be formed just by exposing an unstructured blob of neural material to a succession of stimuli.

The facts are that there *is* a considerable amount of structure that can be found consistently in brain after brain. But there is also evidence of a variability that cannot be attributed to genetic differences. Recently Cyrus Levinthal and Eduardo R. Macagno at Columbia University compared structural details in *genetically identical* nervous systems of the freshwater crustacean *Daphnia*. They found that significant differences exist from specimen to specimen in the precise number and location of synapses, although the overall plan remains fixed. Here then is a clear example of microscopic variability in the brain structures of *identical twins*. To call such variable features *random* merely demonstrates our ignorance of the factors that could have led to one structure in one specimen and a different structure in another. The discovery also implied that for the purpose of a healthy, functioning *Daphnia* brain, it makes little difference which particular realization of the general plan is employed. It can be inferred that evolution assumed genetic control over all essential features, leaving to chance those which can be varied with impunity.

Such detailed structural comparisons have not been accomplished for brains of higher animals, but it can hardly be expected that man's brain has less variability than that of the lowly *Daphnia*. Unfortunately, between what is known to be predetermined and what is known to be variable lies a vast territory of structural detail for which the question of determinism or randomness cannot be answered with assurance. We can say, however, that—unless totally new factors determining structure are discovered—a considerable part of the brain's microstructure must be attributable to the myriads of microscopic and submicroscopic *accidents* we lump together and call chance. The resulting random features will then become permanently embedded in the developing brain. At the same time, experience and learning become the fine texture that is laid down on this structure in the course of our lives.

This somewhat lengthy and, to some, probably tedious discussion is necessary to make two important points to which I will return later. The first is that in the mature brain it may be impossible to make a distinction (even in principle) between random characteristics that are native and *acquired* characteristics. The second point concerns the problem of *reading* brain states, mentioned briefly in Chapter 1 in connection with the *neural identity theory*. The question was raised there whether a precise knowledge of the *state* of someone's brain could tell us precisely what his sensations are and what is "on his mind." If the interpretation above is correct, then such detailed reading of the neuronal code may well necessitate, among other things, a knowledge of the structure of that particular brain far beyond what we can reasonably expect any experiment to determine.

There are other aspects of apparent randomness that have less to do with structure than with function. Functional indeterminacy takes many forms. It is known that individual neurons in a sensory system —the visual system, for example—emit a continuous stream of action potentials even if there is no visual input. Such *spontaneous activity* follows no predictable pattern and must be considered random by our criteria. Given this background of random firings throughout much of the nervous system, it is difficult to maintain that the dynamics of any part of the system can be predicted in detail. Indeed, when the responses of a single neuron to precisely controlled identical stimuli are compared, we find that the precise temporal sequences of action potentials are never the same.

I started this discussion with a quote from Palay, one of the strongest statements of faith in the *necessity* of precise neural circuitry, and I will end it with a quote from Jacques Monod. This passage does not refer directly to the role of chance in neural circuitry, but rather to the alternatives of chance and design (or necessity) in the origin of life. Concerning the idea of a chance origin, Monod states:

> Not only for scientific reasons do biologists recoil at this idea. It runs counter to our very human tendency to believe that behind everything real in the world stands a necessity rooted in the very beginning of things. Against this notion, this powerful feeling of destiny, we must be constantly on guard. Immanence is alien to modern science. Destiny is written concurrently with the event, not prior to it.[7]

But can we really draw the line between chance and necessity? Is chance merely a crutch for which the scientist reaches when all else fails? And is perhaps the gulf between the determinists and the randomizers more semantic than real? I will return to these questions in Chapter 6.

Nature and nurture

If we look back at the early pictorial representations of the brain, we find that generally there is some space set aside whose specific function is the storage of past events: the *memory*. In Reisch's famous drawing (Fig. 2.3, page 40) it was the last of the ventricles. By coincidence the artificial brains, our electronic computers, invented several centuries later, conform quite well to this notion. The heart of the computer, after the *central processing unit*, is a *central* or *core memory*. This consists of banks of many thousands of tiny elements that can be set and reset like so many little switches. Here is where the computer keeps data and constants used in computations, intermediate results, and the programs and subroutines that are the *acquired skills* of the computer. In addition, there is *peripheral* memory storage in devices such as magnetic tapes or disks, where additional programs, too bulky for the core memory, are kept along with the often voluminous data produced by the computer.

Peripheral storage in a computer can be compared to the external memory devices man has been using for millennia: reference libraries, and logs and notebooks into which new material can be deposited. In human as in computer memory, the internal or *core* memory is limited in volume, but has the advantage of being readily accessible. The *reading* of peripheral memory, like the search for a library reference or a word in a dictionary, is very slow by comparison. There are many other close and attractive analogies between brains and computers. It is understandable, therefore, that in trying to understand the brain, we frequently look for suggestions in our most elaborate brainchild, the computer.

The term *memory* implies that something in the brain has changed as a result of events perceived in the past. This physical record is sometimes called the *engram*. The idea that experience *writes* on an initially blank page, a *tabula rasa,* goes back to Aristotle. Today we no longer believe that we bring so little into the world with us, although the relative proportions of *nature* and *nurture* in our personalities are still a matter of dispute among psychologists.

Before discussing what little we know about the mechanisms and the location of memory in the brain, let us look at the equally obscure processes by which the developing embryonic brain organizes itself and reaches the state at which learning can commence.

The prenatal brain consists of more or less disjointed populations of neurons which send out bundles of axons that invade other populations and make synaptic contacts. It has recently been established that the structure which the mammalian brain possesses around the time of birth comes about after a series of false starts. Neurons are not formed in the embryo in the places where they will eventually function but must migrate to their proper destinations. What guides this process is not known, but mistakes are made and cells frequently find themselves in the wrong locations. Most of these so-called *ectopic* cells disappear later during embryonic development. The number of neurons is much too high in some parts of the embryonic brain. This too is corrected by subsequent cell death. As many as 75 percent of the neurons present in some structures die before birth. Many of the connections made initially turn out to be wrong or at least inappropriate. These too are corrected. Synaptic junctions are established in great numbers and then again abandoned. Often there is an initial overproduction of synapses followed by the elimination of the unwanted ones. It is almost as if an electronics engineer were to construct a radio or a TV set by putting together an overabundant supply of transistors and other circuit components, and connecting everything to everything. To achieve a functioning device, the engineer then takes a pair of wire cutters, judiciously snips all the unwanted connections, and deletes all the superfluous components.

We don't know why construction of the brain proceeds in that manner, or what controls all these processes. But we do know that at no stage is the brain the blank page Aristotle thought it was. A modern version of Aristotle's idea is the theory that the brain is a formless mass of neurons at the outset, and that somehow the stream of experience impinging on it gradually shapes it into a feeling, knowing, and planning instrument. The process held responsible for this extraordinary development is called *self-organization.*

There are, of course, many features that emerge as we learn. Language is one of them. But even here the *disposition* to talk is certainly an inherited characteristic of humans. Noam Chomsky goes farther than that. He believes that the common structures of all human languages point to genetic factors controlling the structure. Also very specific areas in the left hemisphere of the human neocortex are set aside for speech, and injuries in these areas generally cause irreparable damage to our ability to use language. But—and there is always a *but* which makes this controversy so persistent—the speech area is part of that remarkably homogeneous mass of neurons, the *isocortex*. To confuse the issue further, other regions of the neocortex are able to assume the function of the speech area if the latter is injured very early in life.

At any rate, to say that the brain is entirely the product of self-organizing processes is to disregard a large body of facts. We start at birth with a functioning, highly differentiated brain. It controls all our vital functions and has a wide repertory of innate behavioral responses. But, just as important, it has an enormous capacity to absorb, to store, to be modified through learning. This capacity is coupled with an eagerness, a powerful drive to learn, to explore, to be invaded by experience. *Innate in the brain?*

It is generally agreed that most of our learning takes place in the neocortex, although significant changes connected with learning may take place in other brain structures. However, many skills once thought to be acquired through learning turn out to be native; that is, they are part of the genetically determined structure and function of the brain. Some maturing of the appropriate parts of the nervous or muscular systems may be required. The fledgling bird does not *learn* to fly from its parents as was once believed; at most, they may urge him on. It was discovered that without the parental example flying is accomplished at the normal time and with the same average success rate. Nor is there a chance to practice. The first flight, requiring precise timing among the neurons that control many different muscles, must be successful. There is no second chance.

In vertebrates the spinal cord is a repository of many elaborate programs of muscle action, especially those pertaining to locomotion. As in the case of bird flight, most of these are probably innate. A study of how these programs are laid down in the neural networks of the spinal cord, and how they are read out, may tell us what kind of organization is required for *learned* behavior. In other words, the *acquired* neural mechanisms inherent in a violinist's trill are perhaps similar to those innate mechanisms that govern the beating of a bird's wing. Unfortunately, we know very little about either.

If memory is a physical thing, it must have a location. In 1926 Karl S. Lashley, a young physiological psychologist at the Institute for Juvenile Research in Chicago, set out methodically to track down the seat of memory. His approach was two-pronged. Working with rats, he surgically removed various portions of their cerebral cortices either before or after the rats had learned certain tasks. In the first case he had hoped to locate the structures responsible for learning, in the second the location of the stored information. The experiments extended over almost a quarter of a century and terminated with his now famous paper, "In Search of the Engram," in 1950.[8]

Lashley did not find the location of the engram, nor that of the learning mechanism. Instead his experiments showed that destruction of almost any part of the neocortex would *dim* the memory of a given learned task. The more extensive the damage, the poorer the performance. The same was true for the ability to learn new tasks. The case must not be overstated, however. There are brain areas with well-defined functions, such as the speech center. Also every sensory input to the neocortex arrives at a sensory area set aside specifically for that *modality*, not at a *common sensorium* as the early anatomists thought.

But for most complex tasks, those involving perhaps several different senses, Lashley found a discouraging *equipotentiality*: Every part of the neocortex contributed a little, and one part contributed about as much as another. He concluded that any single event must involve the activity of perhaps millions of neurons scattered over the neocortex. His fruitless search for the engram made him remark that memory really should not be possible.

The idea of a *distributed memory* has been the prevalent view since Lashley. It gained in popularity especially after the invention of the laser hologram in the early sixties. In this technique, light from a laser is used to record a scene on photographic film. This is called a *hologram* (see Fig. 3.4). Unlike the photographic images taken by an ordinary camera, the hologram itself reveals nothing to the beholder. The film is covered evenly by fine irregular ripples called *interference fringes*. Only when the hologram is again illuminated with laser light through a particular optical system will the original scene be recreated. What appears now is seen fully in three dimensions as though it were the original object standing in space. The viewer can literally walk around it and look at it, or even photograph it from different directions (Fig. 3.5).

There are two other remarkable things about holograms. One is that any small portion of the film on which the information is stored can be used to reproduce the entire scene. The smaller the portion used, the fuzzier will be the final image. But no part of the image is cut off when the hologram is cut. Information about every part of the scene, it turns

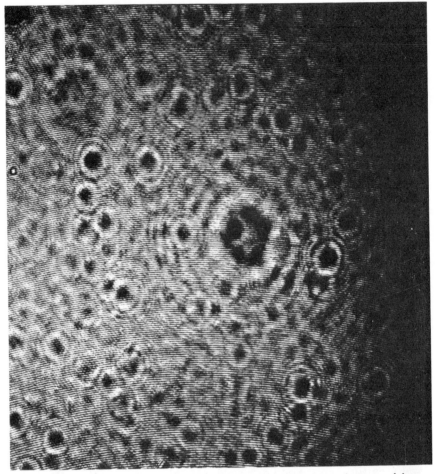

3.4 *A hologram. The fine irregular ripples, called interference fringes, reveal nothing of the scene contained in the image.*

out, is distributed over the entire area of the hologram. What interests brain theorists about the hologram is this quality of a *distributed memory:* Every piece of the hologram says a little bit about every part of the scene, but no piece is essential. The other intriguing fact is that one can superimpose any number of holograms on the same piece of film, and then reproduce the images of the original scenes one by one without interference from the others. The analogy with Lashley's neocortex was all too obvious, and soon theorists began to talk seriously about a *holographic theory of memory.* It has even been suggested that the whole world is a hologram. While some scientists still believe that the processes of memory formation are very similar to those involved in

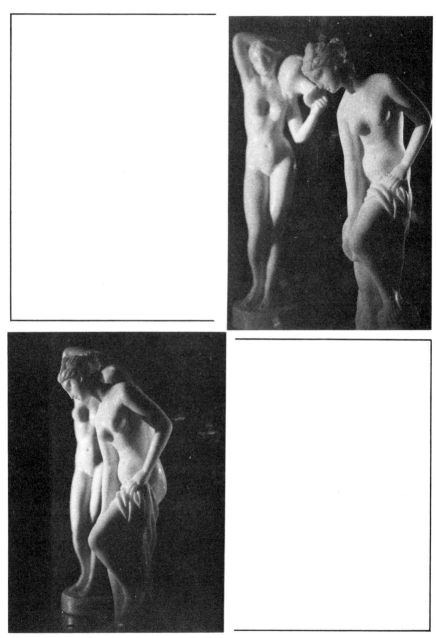

3.5 *Two views (taken with an ordinary camera) of the reconstructed three-dimensional scene contained in a hologram such as the one shown in Fig. 3.4. (From* Optical Holography, *R. J. Collier, C. B. Burckhardt, and L. H. Lin, Academic Press, New York, N.Y., 1971)*

holography, others think that the analogy has only superficial significance.[9]

What then is the nature of the engrams? We know little more than that they are distributed. What has been done to the network of neurons to make them act differently after learning has taken place? There are a number of good guesses but few facts.

As a general guideline, we can take what W. Ritchie Russell calls the "physiological basis of memory and learning", that is, the capacity of the neural system to *repeat*, or the fact that "what has been done before can more easily be done again."[10]

A powerful theory that has dominated thinking along these lines was proposed by Donald O. Hebb in 1949.[11] According to Hebb, patterns of neural activity coursing through the network become *fixed*, or *entrained*, by the strengthening of the synaptic junctions between the neurons involved. The more a particular junction is used or *activated*, the stronger it becomes. This process is called *synaptic facilitation*. As a result, a particular pattern, once established and learned, can easily be refreshed in the future. Hebb called the *constellations* of neurons involved in such reexcitation *cell assemblies*. We can think of different cell assemblies as being associated with different sensory events, or even with different abstract concepts.

It is conceivable that all our learning is based on this single principle of synaptic facilitation. To explore this idea many brain theorists have done extensive calculations or tests using large electronic computers. Such *computer simulations* are not equivalent to demonstrating the existence of the effect in living tissue, but they are valuable in testing whether an idea has a chance of being correct. In one such study Erich Harth and Stacey Edgar[12] showed that associative memory, brought about through synaptic facilitation, can account for a variety of cognitive tasks. In a network containing about a thousand neuron-like elements, different groups of neurons were arbitrarily assigned different meanings as if they were Hebbian cell assemblies. One can think of one such group as representing the object PENCIL, another, FIRE ENGINE, a third, TRAFFIC SIGN. Three other cell assemblies stand for the colors RED, YELLOW, and BLUE, and a fourth for the concept COLOR. Another set represents the materials WOOD, METAL, and PLASTIC, and the concept MATERIAL.

Associations were made by turning on pairs of such cell assemblies —for example, PENCIL and YELLOW—and strengthening all the synapses linking these cell groups. In this way the network was *taught*

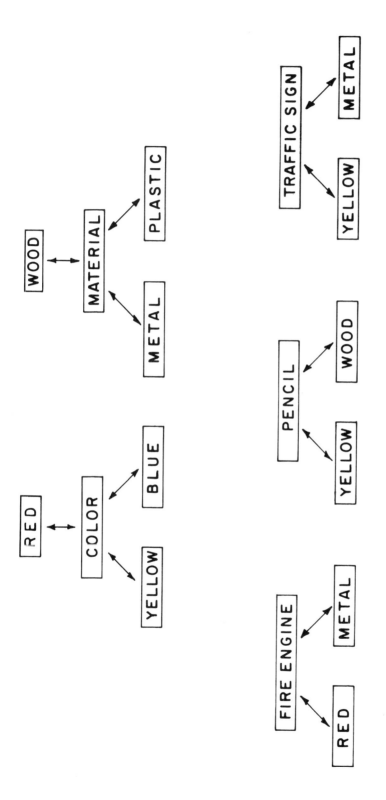

3.6 *Computer simulation of associations made during teaching a neural network*

that pencils are yellow and fire engines red; that wood is a material and blue is a color; and so forth. These association pairs are shown by the double arrows in Fig. 3.6.

Following this teaching phase, the network exhibits something like a primitive intelligent behavior. When the cell assemblies corresponding to YELLOW and WOOD are stimulated, the activity overflows into the assembly corresponding to PENCIL. We can think of the input as a question ("What is WOOD and YELLOW?") and the output as the answer ("PENCIL"). When the network gives no answer, a question mark is shown in the answer column. Thus the network sees nothing similar between FIRE ENGINE and PENCIL, but reminds us that FIRE ENGINE and TRAFFIC SIGN are both METAL, and that PENCIL and TRAFFIC SIGN are both YELLOW. The table on page 93 lists the questions (Q) put to our network and the answers (A) suggested by the neural activity produced.

This somewhat dim-witted brain, if we can call it that, has never heard of any wooden object that is red, or of anything made out of plastic of *any* color. But it does know that plastic and metal are materials, and it will tell you the correct color of a traffic sign. Note also that there remains a logical order to the associations. Thus while the inputs METAL and RED produce FIRE ENGINE, no answer results from FIRE ENGINE and RED.

Like the brain but unlike any computer, the network has a memory that is distributed, and the processing of information proceeds in a parallel rather than a serial fashion. To the question "What is metal and yellow?" the computer would first produce a list of all known metal objects (fire engines and traffic signs) and then eliminate all those that are not yellow. Our neural network, by contrast, uses the two cues "METAL" and "YELLOW", for which there is one immediate reaction, "TRAFFIC SIGN."

The main purpose of the experiment was to test the idea that information may be stored in a network of neurons and remain accessible, using only the principle of synaptic facilitation. It should be pointed out that the associative memory built into our neural network has these three properties of real brains which seemed so analogous to holograms: (1) Memory is distributed over most of the network; (2) any position of the network will reproduce the entire engram, but the clarity of the reproduction depends on the portion of the network used; (3) different engrams can be superimposed on the same space and be

Q:		A:
(What is the)_____	**(of a)_____(?)**	
MATERIAL	FIRE ENGINE	METAL
COLOR	FIRE ENGINE	RED
MATERIAL	PENCIL	WOOD
COLOR	PENCIL	YELLOW
MATERIAL	TRAFFIC SIGN	METAL
COLOR	TRAFFIC SIGN	YELLOW
(What is)_____	**(and)_____(?)**	
METAL	RED	FIRE ENGINE
METAL	YELLOW	TRAFFIC SIGN
METAL	BLUE	?
WOOD	RED	?
WOOD	YELLOW	PENCIL
WOOD	BLUE	?
PLASTIC	RED	?
PLASTIC	YELLOW	?
PLASTIC	BLUE	?
(What is common between)_____	**(and)_____(?)**	
FIRE ENGINE	PENCIL	?
FIRE ENGINE	TRAFFIC SIGN	METAL
PENCIL	TRAFFIC SIGN	YELLOW
(What are)_____	**(and)_____(?)**	
BLUE	YELLOW	COLOR
BLUE	RED	COLOR
RED	YELLOW	COLOR
METAL	WOOD	MATERIAL
METAL	PLASTIC	MATERIAL
PLASTIC	WOOD	MATERIAL

read out individually. It is perhaps significant also that the number of questions the network can answer (seventeen) is greater than the number of associative pairs (twelve) required to train it.

This experiment is one of many performed by different investigators in recent years. It would be foolish to claim that this tells us how the brain works. The theory of synaptic facilitation has a strange built-in flaw: It works too well! A network of real neurons, or neurons simulated on a computer, with adjustable synaptic junctions has been called a *universal machine*. This means that it can carry out just about any logical task we can think up for it. It is no longer a question of whether an artificial network can do a certain task but how efficiently or how cleverly. Whether the real brain mechanisms conform to our ideas of efficiency and cleverness is anyone's guess.

A discussion of memory storage in the brain would not be complete without some mention of an entirely different approach which became popular a number of years ago. Analogies again played a role here. This time a connection was sought with two other types of memory. *Genetic memory* is carried by the molecules of DNA which every living cell inherits and passes on to its offspring. The message here consists of a long string of letters, the *nucleotides* of which DNA is composed. Another type of memory is the *immune response*. It is not nearly as well understood as genetic memory, but it is also known to be molecular in character. Our bodies manufacture certain proteins— the *immunoglobulins*, or *antibodies*. Each type of antibody is specific to a particular irritant, or *antigen*, to which we have been exposed. These antigens can be anything from an influenza virus, to a foreign histocompatibility antigen from an organ transplant, to a simple chemical to which we have become allergic. The antibodies we carry in our system are thus the *immunological memory* of the invasions our bodies have suffered in the past.

This evident ability of organic molecules to acquire, retain, and yield complex information was taken by some to be a hint that the memories held in our brains may be of similar character. This viewpoint was strengthened when in the early sixties Holger Hydén in Sweden reported changes in the amount and character of ribonucleic acids (RNA) in neurons after they had been subjected to intense activity. Soon RNA was hailed by some scientists as the *memory molecule*. At about the same time, several investigators announced that learning could be facilitated and memory actually transferred from one animal to another by injecting brain extracts or simply by letting an untrained animal eat and digest one that has learned a certain task. The experiments were done first with flatworms and later with mice. Jokes abounded about students eating their professors to gain knowledge. We know, of course, that certain cannibalistic tribes believe the strength and the bravery of a victim are acquired by the one who eats him.

More recently scientists who tried to repeat the flatworm experiments obtained mostly negative results. A passionate controversy ensued, showing that science is not always the smooth progression of knowledge that scientists like to picture to the layman. Eventually the molecular theory of memory fell into disfavor. At a recent conference dedicated to the investigation of memory mechanisms, not one of the many papers presented was in support of the molecular theory.

Chance into essence

Let us pull together some of the facts and some of the guesses from the last sections. The human neocortex contains tens of billions of neurons, each of which makes thousands of connections with other neurons. These are the synapses, some ten or a hundred trillion of them, whose strengths and precise distribution determine the precise dynamic properties of the brain. We must always bear in mind the vastness of this structure and the mass of minute detail it contains. A structural determinist would argue that nothing in this network is left to chance.

I have pointed out that it is possible in principle for all the details of the native human brain to be genetically determined, but only if there is a very large amount of symmetry or redundancy in the structure. The variability observed in much more primitive, genetically identical neural structures have led us to believe that many of the details of the neonatal human brain—we don't know how many—are likely to be the product of chance.

Chance certainly plays a role in determining the microstructure of our other organs. But wherever chance appears, or is allowed to appear in the course of the organism's development, its vagaries turn out to be nonessential. Evolution has seen to that, devising strict rules wherever necessary and giving rein to chance only where it can do no harm. I will now argue that in the case of our brain, this nonessential character of chance events is only temporary, and that in the mature brain every minute detail may well play a role, albeit a very minute role. In this sense one can say that every detail is essential.

These arguments, I must stress, are conjectures based first on the assumption of random elements in the formation of our brains, and second on the theory of learning by some sort of modification of the synapses. The first assumption is difficult to prove but equally difficult to avoid. The second is at present still our best bet.

Picture the infant brain at birth, its structure a unique blend of heritage and chance. The information now streaming in along all sensory pathways, and the resulting neural activities, produce subtle changes in the strengths of the trillions of synapses. We believe that memories are formed in this way. But the tablet on which these memories are written is rough—at first only with the meaningless accidental bumps present from birth, but soon also with the imprints of millions of fleeting sense impressions too faint to be called memories.

The picture I am trying to convey here has two interesting aspects I want to emphasize once again. The early effects of chance, frozen into the infant brain as part of the permanent microstructure, become the stuff from which memories will be sculpted. Thus chance is turned into essence. The inverse processes also occur. The weakest of the sense impressions recede into the background, becoming part of and indistinguishable from the texture of the neural network. If this is a correct picture, then chance and necessity, randomness and structure meld into one in the human brain. No logical distinctions can be drawn between these properties. The brain is perhaps the only structure for which this is true. This feature is a guarantee of absolute uniqueness of every brain, even those belonging to identical twins.

Neurophysiologists often talk of a *neural code*, implying there may be some general, as yet undiscovered method of relating what goes on inside the head to what goes on outside. An analogy can be drawn again from molecular biology. Sequences of nucleotides in the DNA molecule specify the structures of proteins the organism produces. The translation of one into the other is called the *genetic code*. Since this code was broken in 1966, scientists have been able to *read* sections of DNA molecules and learn what sequence of amino acids is called for in the construction of protein. The code, it turns out, is *universal*: Every organism living on earth uses the same language. A section of DNA from a mammal inserted into the DNA of a bacterium such as *E. coli* will cause the bacterium's protein factory to produce the same protein that would have been manufactured by the mammal. This is the basis of recombinant DNA technology, or *genetic engineering*.

By contrast, it seems unlikely that anything like a universal *neural code* exists in the nervous system. If memories are distributed over many synapses, and if the original structure contains a substantial amount of randomness, then the neural activity that goes with a particular mental act will be very different for different brains. Transmitting the pattern of such activity from one brain to another, if it could be done, would only produce meaningless babble. The meaning of neural activity is probably not even fixed for a particular individual but is a dynamic function. The code thus appears elusive, undecipherable, and we would do better to not even speak of a neural code except perhaps for the periphery of the nervous system.

Neurons in the mammalian brain do not regenerate. They have lost this valuable talent, or what Monod has called "the dream of every cell: to become two cells." Why? I will indulge in one more guess here. If it is true that the early work of chance has become essence in the mature brain, then no regrowth of brain matter can restore what has been lost due to injury, disease, or age. Chance cannot be re-created. A nervous system that is for the most part determined by genetic blueprints can be regenerated as long as the blueprint is preserved. In lower vertebrates this type of regeneration is readily observed. It appears that the loss of this ability is the price we mammals have to pay for a brain which is designed to be the repository of a unique selfhood that arises when chance is molded into essence.

4

A VIEW FROM BELOW

Only a creature that acts is capable of knowing.

—CARL I. LEWIS

Where thoughts are made

In our exploration up to now, we have been following a classic pattern of seeking a summit and stopping on the way only long enough to ask which way is up. Warren McCullough once wrote an article entitled "Why the Mind Is in the Head."[1] His point was quite simply that this is the only place where structure is complex enough to account for higher brain functions.

But aren't we perhaps a little like the comic visitor from another planet with his stereotyped command "Take me to your leader?" His stratagem would of course be appropriate unless he happened to have landed in a participatory democracy, in which case he would earn only ridicule and wind up in a cartoon. Not unlike this character, we have been expecting a tightly ruled, hierarchic society of neurons, but may have stumbled instead into a democracy that is both heterogeneous in structure and diffuse of purpose. We must now descend from the elitist neocortex and reassess the role of the hardworking peripheral neurons.

At a seminar I once tried to make the point that thoughts are not just rumblings in the cortex but often involve the nervous system at all levels. I asked members of the audience to think of their favorite tactile fantasy. Soon scores of fingers began to wriggle surreptitiously, showing that not all of the mind is in the head. (I have referred before to the very real sensations produced by the mere thought of fingernails scratching across a blackboard.) It is possible of course that these peripheral activities are only by-products, tremors sent down from the highest brain centers, spillovers from overactive minds.

This raises crucial questions: Where are thoughts made? Where do we initiate the processes of thinking about something? And where do we proceed to spin out thoughts, manipulate images, play with imagined sense perceptions as if they were real, react to them with actions of our own, except that these two are mostly "in our minds"? There are two prevalent views on this question. One is that these transactions are confined to the highest domain, perhaps the frontal lobes of the cortex, away from the areas assigned to specific senses or motor actions. According to the other view, images are like "weak sense perceptions," which they mimic, and they originate somewhere in the sensory pathways. The question is by no means settled, and good arguments are adduced on both sides. Several factors cause me to favor the second view or some variation thereof. One is the observation that by itself the neocortex—for all its complexity and its exalted position in the brain—is incapable of thought. Even when properly supplied with all its necessary nutrients *and* a normal inflow of sensory information, it would languish in a deep coma unless it interacted with other brain structures. The one structure without which consciousness cannot exist is called the *reticular activating system,* or RAS, which is in the brainstem. A permanently damaged RAS means irreversible coma. By contrast, even extensive damage in the cortex, through accident or surgery, will not impair consciousness, as we saw in the example of Phineas Gage. It was shown also in the extensive surgical experience reported by the late Canadian neurosurgeon Wilder Penfield that no single portion of the cortex is essential for conscious activity. It is difficult to reconcile these facts with the picture of an autonomous thinking center in the cortex.

Another reason for reexamining the role of the neocortex is a phenomenon psychologists call *projection.* This is a somewhat vague and controversial concept. It has to do with the fact that an external event, picked up by our senses, is *felt* not at the final destination of the flow of signals but at their source. We hear the bell ring in the bell tower, not in our head. The puzzle of projection, indeed the puzzle of *percep-*

tion, is that a *neural event* in the brain appears as a happening outside the body. We have no feeling of where in our head neural relays are being tripped, hence we do not know from direct experience what parts of the brain are engaged in a particular activity. Instead we point infallibly to the sources of sense perceptions in the outside world.

There is a curious parallel to this type of spatial *projection,* namely, a referral of consciousness *backward in time.*

William James, in *Principles of Psychology,* refers to this phenomenon. "Perception," he says, "seems to be retrospective and the time order of events to be read off in memory rather than known at the moment."[2]

Consciousness, it turns out, is a slow phenomenon. We will discuss in Chapter 5 some experiments by Benjamin Libet which strongly suggest that about half a second elapses before we can become conscious of an event our senses have picked up. This is a long time, considering it takes only a few hundredths of a second for a stimulus to go from peripheral sensors—for example, touch receptors in the skin—to the cortex, and about a tenth of a second to react with some predetermined motor act to an anticipated event.

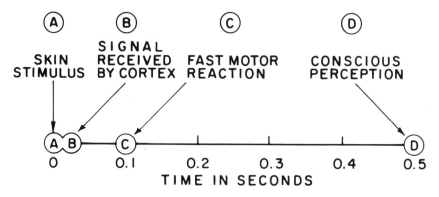

4.1 *Consciousness of a sensory event. A touch to the skin occurs at A and is signaled to the cortex at B. At C the subject is able to react, for example, by pressing a button. He will, however, not be* conscious *of the sensation nor of his own reaction, until the instant marked D. Nevertheless, he feels that C was a* conscious *act.*

In Fig. 4.1 four events are shown on a time scale marked off in tenths of a second. At A, a touch stimulus is applied to the skin. The first action potentials signaling the event arrive in the cortex as early as ten milliseconds later (point B). If the subject is told beforehand to push a button as soon as he feels the skin stimulus, he may react in about one tenth of a second. This is point C. But conscious knowledge of the stimulus does not occur until point D in the figure, about half a second later. At that time we are not only conscious of A and C, but we are also convinced that the act C was a conscious response to the event A. Thus the delayed consciousness is *referred back* to the instant the event occurred.

Our brain, it appears, falsifies both the location and time of neural events, thereby placing our cognitive selves *out there*, where and when the real events are happening, and making us feel almost independent of all that cumbersome machinery in our heads. This belies the classical notion of a conscious self that is enclosed in the sightless, soundless, and odorless world of the brain capsule, receiving news only in coded form about the sights, sounds, and smells of the world. The immediacy of our sensations as well as the inability of the isolated cortex to sustain consciousness suggest that the boundaries of consciousness extend well beyond the braincase, probably to the very surface of the body and even beyond. Niels Bohr has made the point that the boundary of our observing self is not even rigidly drawn. "We cannot even tell which particular molecules belong to a living organism."[3] Also, a pencil held tightly can become an extension of one's tactile sensors: It conveys the texture and unevenness of the surface over which it is drawn. But when held loosely, the same pencil is part of the outside world, sensed by the tips of one's fingers.

A very similar thought was expressed several centuries earlier by Leonardo da Vinci in a discourse on the anatomy of the nervous system. "The hand that holds the stone within it when it is struck with a hammer," says Leonardo, "feels part of the pain which the stone would feel if it were a sentient body."[4] It should be remarked here that the participation of peripheral parts of the nervous system in shaping our knowledge of the world has never been in doubt. We need our eyes to see, our fingers to palpate, and so forth. On the output side of the nervous system we need our effectors, chiefly our muscles, to act on the outside world.

This picture is simple enough and conforms very nicely to the scheme presented in Fig. 2.8 on page 47, which shows receptors on one side, the afferent side, and effectors on the other. But such a brain would have few human qualities. It lacks the ability to *pretend*, to try out patterns of sensations and actions by simulating them. That such simulations cannot take place wholly in isolation seems evident from the fact that true sensations and fantasies come in all mixes, from the *almost* objective observations of a scientist who carries out an experiment to full-blown hallucinations. For the intermediate cases there must be a lively exchange between sensory fact and stored fact, between imagined sensation and imagined action, the expected and the perceived.

The neural mechanisms responsible for these transactions are mostly obscure, but most involve pathways that run counter to the prevalent stream of neural information flow. On the afferent side we find fibers going from the cortex *to* the periphery, certainly as far as the thalamus, and in some animals they go all the way back to the receptors. Unlike the simple diagram shown in Fig. 2.8, the sensory pathways are not unidirectional but form loops whereby the simulating, conjecturing, confabulating cortex can influence the stream of incoming information.

The word *reflection* appears in this context to be a very apt description of *thought*. The cortex literally reflects, bounces back images that have impinged on it, producing new and modified inputs for itself. At the same time, it may send messages down motor pathways and play with the sensory echoes of such simulated actions.

But as soon as we give up unidirectionality on either the afferent or efferent side of the brain, we also forsake the concept of strict neuronal hierarchy. The cerebral cortex appears not so much a summit as a *hub* of many intersecting loops.

Returning once again to the question "Where are thoughts made?", readers are aware by now that I do not favor the notion of a self-contained "thinking cap." The seeds of thought may spring up anywhere in the nervous system, but a fully developed thought requires more than the neocortex. Thinking is a *bootstrap* mechanism. It may be as absurd to expect thought from a brain without an attached body as it would be to expect consciousness from a body without a brain.

I should make clear that this point of view is not shared by all neuroscientists. Michael Gazzaniga of Cornell University Medical College in New York City believes that "mental life is transacted in codes that transcend perceptual experience on the neural level," and that "the neural mechanisms that have evolved for transacting business with the external world (i.e., perceptual-motor mechanisms) are not the mechanisms by which we conduct our mental life."[5]

In the remainder of this chapter we will take a closer look at some selected portions of the nervous system. We will discuss vision, the most exquisite of the sensory systems, and pain, the most baffling one. We will *look up* into the brain, first from the sensory, then from the motor side, and see where the two systems join: the *central sulcus*. But first we will ask how it all came about.

How brains are made

The search for the brain's origins can take two distinct paths. We can examine the nervous systems of our ancestors along the evolutionary ladder all the way back to the most primitive life forms, or we can trace the development of the brain in the individual from the fertilized ovum, through the embryonic and fetal stages, to infancy and on to maturity. We can hope that the simplicity we find in either the primordial or the rudimentary forms will aid our understanding of the functioning of the mature human brain.

The two paths are quite different. In one we find the rules of evolution operating over hundreds of millions of years and involving vast populations of individuals, each measuring for a brief span the fitness of its body—and especially the keenness of its nervous system—against the rigors of its environment. Slowly evolution filters the most efficient designs out of the passing populations. The process is so slow that only in a few exceptional cases have we been able to observe the natural change of a species during our own lifetime. (Of course, changes brought about through human selection and manipulation are commonplace.) Yet we believe that all the species we know today, and many more that have long ago vanished, were derived from some inchoate ancestor by the rules of the survival of the fittest. In this way evolution gave rise to the multiplicity of life-forms that fill every ecological niche of our planet. Biologists call this process *phylogeny*.

The other route to a primitive brain is much shorter and much more accessible, since we can easily examine the brain at every stage of the embryo. The development of the individual from single cell to maturity is called *ontogeny*, and there is an old adage in biology that says, "Ontogeny recapitulates phylogeny." This means simply that the successive stages of the embryo bear a resemblance to earlier evolutionary forms. Every individual repeats, so to speak, the whole evolutionary process. The statement has a superficial plausibility but very little substance. Evolution, or phylogeny, is traversed only once in all of eter-

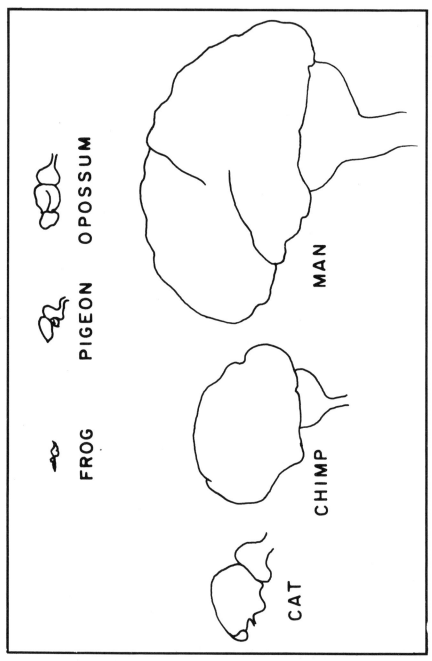

4.2 Evolution of the vertebrate nervous system. The brains of living vertebrates are drawn to the same scale. (Redrawn after David H. Hubel)

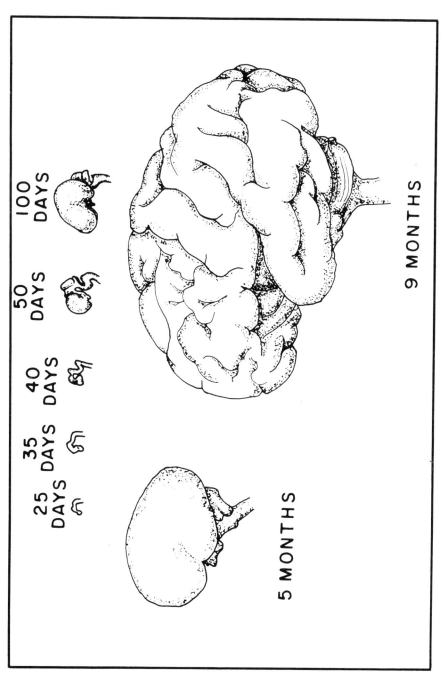

4.3 *Development of the human brain from embryo to birth. (After W. Maxwell Cowan)*

nity, and will continue as long as there is life on the planet. There are no repeats. Every change is new, and the outcome is always unknown. Ontogeny, by contrast, is repeated over and over again, following with minor variations the same path. Healthy infants have predictable forms. The brain of a genius cannot be distinguished from that of an individual of very moderate intelligence.

But a more fundamental difference between the two sequences has to do with the fact that every brain in evolutionary history must have been capable of supporting the organism in its struggle for existence, or else that branch of the evolutionary tree would have ended there. The embryonic brain, by contrast, has less stringent requirements, since the embryo is in a benevolent environment, nourished, and sheltered from adversity.

Evolutionary changes must be gradual, with every intermediate step a viable, functioning system. This is a point we must keep in mind whenever we compare the design of an organ, whether it is a brain or a limb for locomotion, with an engineering solution. The engineer can make an optimal design, then construct and put the system into operation. The design of a living organ must be accessible via a continuous chain of viable and nearly identical models, starting with its most primitive prototype.

The embryonic development is something intermediate between the ongoing engineering done in evolution and the assembly-line construction of a fully designed car or electronic circuit. The embryo must develop from primitive beginnings, but many of its parts don't have to function until the building process is completed. Large parts of the brain, as we shall see, remain nonfunctional for extended periods while they are being assembled according to a predetermined plan.

Our knowledge of the evolution of the brain is sketchy. This is mostly due to the fact that we cannot examine directly the nervous systems of evolutionary ancestors, but must be content to look at primitive but *contemporary* brains. We are aided, of course, by the fossil record, which tells us that many living species are in fact survivors of very early life-forms.

The most primitive animals with a distinguishable nervous system are various types of flatworms, or *Planaria*, of which there are many living representatives. In the lithograph reproduced here (Fig. 4.4), M. C. Escher has captured the arcane character of these creatures. At the same time, the pairs of eyes look at us with a startling familiarity. The pairing of sense organs is a feature that appears at the very begin-

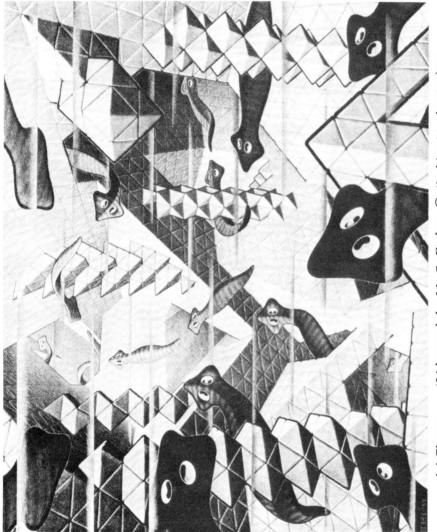

4.4 *Flatworms. (Lithograph by M. C. Escher; © Beeldrecht, Amsterdam, and VAGA, New York. Collection Haags Temeentemuseum)*

ning of the evolution of nervous systems, some 300 million years before the appearance of the first mammals. This bilaterality is reflected in the planarian brain, which shows bilateral bulges, each presumably receiving information from one side of the body and controlling the muscles on that side. Apart from these primitive reflexes, it is believed that the flatworm brain may be capable of retaining some form of memory. A recent symposium on evolution concluded with the remark that "in nature there exists no cyclopean unit brain," and that doubleness with local control for each body half is the "prototype upon which all subsequent nervous systems were developed."[6]

Bilateral symmetry pervades all animal body shapes with few exceptions, a fact that has puzzled biologists and caused some to propose that it results from the dual structure of the basic genetic unit: the double helix of DNA. I think the answer may be simpler than this, and may explain also why automobiles, airplanes, ships, and trains exhibit the same property, and why flying saucers are very unlikely objects. We need only assume that when there is no compelling reason for making it otherwise, the best design is maximal symmetry. Let us start then with the most symmetrical shape, the perfect sphere, and ask why man, locomotive, and kangaroo are not spherical. It becomes immediately obvious that gravity imposes an up-down specialization on all these structures. They must interact with the ground for support, hence they develop on one side special devices, legs or wheels, to accomplish this. The need to move about horizontally further reduces the symmetry. We might, of course, have a shape like the ideal flying saucer, which has a top and a bottom, but no front or rear. This would require a mechanism of propulsion that works equally well in all directions, a fact claimed to have been observed by some flying-saucer buffs. The engineering difficulties to accomplish this are severe and totally unnecessary. It is much simpler to specialize for motion in one direction, with perhaps a less efficient system for occasionally going in reverse. To go anywhere, it is then necessary only to reorient the vehicle and use the unidirectional forward drive. Thus necessity has led us in a natural way from the sphere to a shape that looks different from the top and the bottom, and from front and rear. We have arrived at bilateral symmetry.

One of the persistent features of the evolution of vertebrates is the addition of new structures at the head end of the nervous system. Eventually three distinct parts are formed at the top of the spinal column: the *hindbrain,* the *midbrain,* and the *forebrain* (see Fig. 4.5).

FOREBRAIN   **HINDBRAIN**
MIDBRAIN

SPINAL CORD

4.5 *Three parts of a vertebrate brain formed by a neural tube*

These structures further subdivide and proliferate, but are recognizable in all vertebrate brains. They are formed out of the fundamental embryonic structure of all vertebrate brains, the *neural tube*. The "forward growth" of the nervous system is accompanied by a shifting of functions from older to newer structures. This means that a particular part of the brain which at one stage of evolution carried out a certain set of functions, will at a subsequent stage be confined to the more primitive of these functions. The rest have been passed on to higher brain centers. The forward growth and the upward shift in functions are part of what is called *encephalization*. This process reaches its highest expression in man's brain where the latest and topmost structure, the neocortex, dwarfs all other structures by its sheer size and handles the bulk of all sensory-motor functions.

The following account of the embryonic development of the brain relies heavily on the work of W. Maxwell Cowan of Washington University School of Medicine in St. Louis, with special emphasis on his two review articles on the subject[7], and a series of brilliant lectures delivered in the summer of 1979 in Erice, Sicily.

Cowan distinguishes eight stages in the formation of the brain. Early in the life of the embryo a patch of cells in its outer layer, the *ectoderm*, becomes transformed into specialized tissue which will eventually form the brain. This patch, now "irreversibly committed" to the task of forming the nervous system, is called the *neural plate*. The process is called *induction* because the cells are *induced* to undergo this transformation presumably by some chemical signal coming from below, from the underlying *mesoderm*.

Cells in the neural plate at first have equal potentialities. If a small part of the neural plate is removed from the embryo, the loss will be made up by other cells, and a normal nervous system will develop. At a somewhat later stage, however, the cells of the neural plate become further differentiated to form what will become the forebrain, midbrain, hindbrain, and spinal cord. The differentiation proceeds in that order, with the cells destined to become forebrain specializing first. If any part of the neural plate is excised now, permanent damage will result in the corresponding brain structure. With induction completed, the neural plate, consisting of some 125,000 cells, folds into a cylindrical structure, the *neural tube*.

In the second stage of development the cells of the neural tube begin to divide rapidly and proliferate. The tube becomes multilayered, and the bulk of the billions of cells that will make up the brain are formed. The tissue does not yet act like a nervous system. There are no synaptic connections, no fibers to conduct nervous impulses from one place to another.

In stage three some of the cells lose their ability to divide further and begin to migrate toward the surface of the tube. At this point the neural tube is a thick-walled, somewhat squashed cylinder, shown in Fig. 4.6 in cross section. The region near the central canal, or *ventricle*, is where most of the cell proliferation takes place. Specialized brain cells, the radial *glial cells,* have fibers that reach radially outward from the ventricle to the surface of the neural tube. The young neurons apparently use the glial fibers as their guides in their migration to the

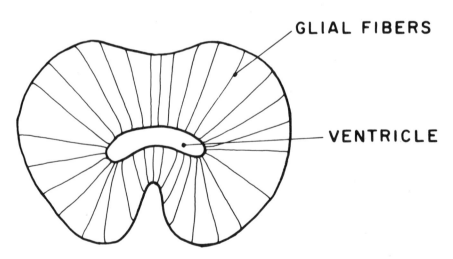

4.6 *Cross section through a neural tube. The radial lines are fibers of glial cells along which migrating neurons will travel. (After W. Maxwell Cowan)*

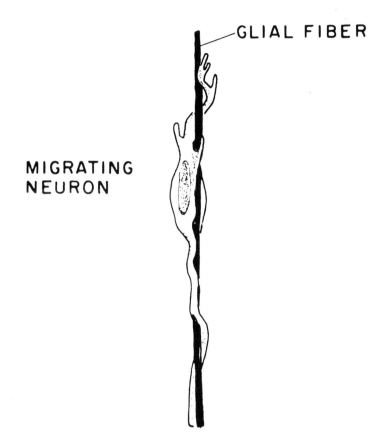

4.7 *Glial fiber with migrating neuron. (After W. Maxwell Cowan)*

place in the brain where they will eventually function. Figure 4.7 is a sketch of one such fiber (black) and a neuron (white) in the process of migration. It shows the neuron using its own processes to adhere to the glial fiber and climb it, like a monkey climbing a rope.

Figure 4.6 is, of course, drastically oversimplified. The neural tube soon becomes a maze of fibers and cell groups that are migrating or have arrived at their destination. The fiber network, in particular, which is composed of processes from glial cells and neurons, soon becomes so dense and intricate that it is justly called a *feltwork*. Migrating neurons must find their way through this maze and arrive at their appropriate locations. One of the fundamental puzzles of brain formation at this stage is how neurons find their way, assuming their destinations are preordained. There is convincing evidence that the glial fibers provide guides for at least some of the wandering neurons. But this only shifts the locus of the puzzle. We must ask then how the glial fibers know in which direction to point, and as yet there is no answer to this question.

If the destinations of the migrating neurons are in some way predetermined, it makes sense to ask how detailed is the map that is being followed. Is the precise location of every neuron specified, or only some general arrangement? Also is the determination absolute, or does it allow deviations or even errors?

We can answer only the last of these questions. Mistakes are made occasionally in the traffic control of the migrating neurons. We find neurons definitely misplaced at various embryonic stages. A type that should be in one place has wandered off to the wrong location. They are called *ectopic* neurons. There is, however, a correcting mechanism: By the time of birth most of these lost neurons will have died.

Stage four is called *aggregation*. Migrating groups of cells of one type consolidate, or aggregate, into structures, forming one after another of the recognizable parts in the mature brain: the cortex, the various midbrain structures and nuclei, the hindbrain and its various subdivisions. It is conjectured that some chemical affinity exists between cells of one type, and that this "selective adhesiveness" accounts for the formation of these structures.

The cells within a given part of the brain are now ready to *differentiate*, that is to specialize further in their functional properties. Among other things, the chemical specificity of each cell is determined in this fifth stage of development. This means the cell is assigned a transmitter substance that it will dispense at its axonal endings. Likewise, the transmitter to which it will be sensitive is now determined.

Stage six is perhaps the most delicate and mysterious. The neurons are ready to extend their fibers and link up, making the enormous number of synaptic connections that constitute the neural network. Only now can we speak of a functioning nervous system. Dendrites branch out in their characteristic patterns, and axons thrust out from the cell bodies, branching and often traveling considerable distances through the nervous system before they select their target cells. Afferent fibers from the sense organs, often neatly bundled into cables, invade and make contact with nuclei in the central nervous system. Similarly, efferent fibers connect to neurons in the spinal cord, and these in turn send axons to terminate on muscle fibers which are frequently a considerable distance away.

Again, we must raise the question, What guides the formation of these connections? To what degree of detail is the circuitry predetermined? How much is left to chance? What influence does the environment have on the nascent network?

We have no final answers to any of these questions, but much new information is accumulating. One of the most important discoveries has been the observation of the so-called *growth cones*, which appear at the ends of the neural fibers at this stage (Fig. 4.8). These are small

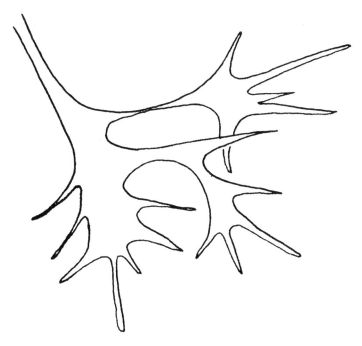

4.8 *Growth cones of a sprouting neural fiber.*

protrusions that reach out, amoeba-like, extending and retracting and seemingly *feeling* their way through the tissue. Movies of growth cones in pieces of living nerve tissue convey this startling impression of an intelligent search, a series of trials and errors, and decision making. They almost seem like bloodhounds sniffing their way through dense underbrush. We must remind ourselves that we are looking here at minute portions of a yet unformed nervous system.

One explanation for the apparent goal-seeking behavior is chemical affinity. This phenomenon, which explains so many effects in biology, may well be the *scent* that guides the searching growth cones to their targets. The theory of chemical labels as the determinants of neural connectivity was first proposed by Roger W. Sperry at the California Institute of Technology in Pasadena. There is some evidence to support this view. Rita Levi-Montalcini of the Laboratory of Cell Biology in Rome, has shown that some axons can be made to follow the route of an injected chemical, the protein NGF (for *nerve growth factor*), which she had discovered earlier.

We come back again and again to the question of how much of the neural circuitry is predetermined, and the precision with which the plan is followed. The reason for this preoccupation is simple: Somewhere in the development of the human brain, genetic factors must be exhausted and individuality must begin; but where?

It is possible, of course, that every single synaptic link is preordained by a chemical marker. This would require many different markers —as well as an enormous amount of genetic information, as discussed earlier (page 78). It is more likely that the chemical markers —or whatever other factors determine the growth of synapses—leave some of the details undecided. There are several features that suggest there is something at least a little haphazard about the way brains are formed. We have already mentioned ectopic cells which wander off to inappropriate places. There are also fibers that go to the wrong target cells and make *ectopic connections*. Apart from these apparent mistakes, there is also an initial overproduction of cells and connections and a subsequent weeding out of superfluous elements.

This selective cell death and the elimination of many previously formed synapses are stages seven and eight, respectively, in the scheme of development described by Cowan. Widespread cell death during embryonic or fetal development is characteristic of many, if not all, parts of the brain. It involves in some regions up to 85 percent of the neural population. Synapse elimination occurs somewhat later and is likely to depend to some extent on functional factors. "The developing brain," says Cowan, "is an extremely plastic structure. Although many regions may be 'hard-wired,' others (such as the cerebral cortex) are open to a variety of influences, both intrinsic and environmental."[8] These "influences" certainly operate on the mechanisms for synapse elimination, and thereby mold the nervous system to deal most efficiently with particular problems and situations encountered early in life.

Recent work shows[9] that the external and internal environments of the nervous system can affect its final form in a variety of ways and at practically all stages of development. Marcus Jacobson of the University of Utah College of Medicine has proposed a theory that neurons such as the pyramidal cells in the cerebral cortex, which are differentiated early in stage five, have rigidly specified connections, whereas the later, small *interneurons* retain the "property of openness."[10] These interneurons are modifiable and will complete the network, according to Jacobson, in ways that reflect the influences of the environment.

E. R. Macagno and coworkers at Columbia University have shown that in the crustacean *Daphnia* neural connections from eyes to brain are modifiable.[11] When the development of the eyes was delayed, the fibers coming from the eye neurons found that their target cells in the brain were already occupied by other fibers. They then made contacts with whatever other cells were still available. In the words of Macagno, "a neuron chooses its friends not because they are especially destined to be its friends, but because they are at the right time and place."

In our discussion of the neocortex (pages 62–68), we pointed to the remarkably uniform structure of this vast neural system, which is in strange contrast to the great variety of specialized functions that different cortical areas support. Unless you are an expert in neuroanatomy, it is not easy to tell from a microphotograph whether you are looking at a section of visual cortex, or somatosensory cortex, or perhaps a part of the speech center.

There are differences, which lie mainly in certain prominent cell types which can be seen to occur in one region but not in another. It seems significant, however, that these differences occur late in the development of the individual, at a time when the afferent and efferent connections are made for each of the cortical regions. It is as though the cortex were able to undergo local modifications according to the processing needs of the peripheral structures to which it is connected. This is again in accordance with Creutzfeldt's belief that the cortex functions as a link between other structures (page 67).

Let us return once more to the evolution of the brain and how it may affect what we are today. We disposed of the old notion that each of us repeats in the womb what had transpired during many hundreds of millions of years of evolution. There is another theory according to which the evolutionary past is still very much with us, even in adult life. According to Paul McLean of the Laboratory of Brain Evolution and Behavior of the National Institutes of Health in Washington, D.C., our brain has evolved in three distinct stages, with each stage building a new superstructure on the previous one.[12] McLean calls these three parts *the reptilian brain* (or R-complex), *the paleomammalian brain,* and *the neomammalian brain.* The human brain, which contains all three of these, he calls *the triune brain* (Fig. 4.9).

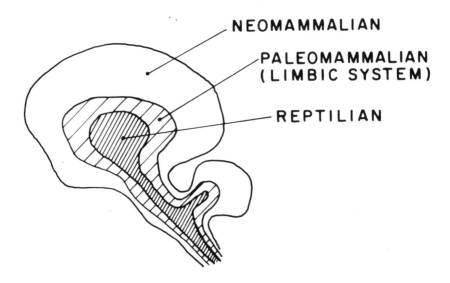

NEOMAMMALIAN

PALEOMAMMALIAN
(LIMBIC SYSTEM)

REPTILIAN

4.9 *The triune brain according to McLean*

In McLean's theory our triune brain resembles an "archeological site," with the reptilian R-complex at the lowest level and the neocortex, our most recent acquisition, near the surface. The lower structures, McLean contends, not only date back to primordial times, but have retained their former functions. He draws parallels between reptilian behavior and corresponding human patterns that he ascribes to the R-complex. There is a *paleopsychology,* he claims, that goes with the R-complex and with the paleomammalian brain. In the colorful language of Arthur Koestler, who describes McLean's work in his book *The Ghost in the Machine,* when a human lies down on a psychiatrist's couch, there are three creatures there: an alligator, a horse, and a man. Koestler goes on to blame many of our social and political ills on a mismatch and the resulting conflicts between our three brain components.

The triune brain is an intriguing theory and has won many advocates. There are critics, however, who point out that functions are interchanged between brain structures during evolution. Similarities in structure and function remain, but no part of the brain remains truly unchanged. McLean's R-complex is unquestionably the oldest part of the brain. But, critics say, it is no longer a reptilian brain, it is simply part of a human brain. McLean's doctrine seems more a point of view than a theory, but perhaps it is instructive, especially in the study of the psychology of human behavior.

The brain of the human newborn leaves the individual almost completely helpless. The system is all there, but it is unable to do what a mature brain does. Sensory-motor coordination is only one of the things that are lacking. More important, the infant brain has yet to develop a whole system of logical structures to connect the world of events with the world of sensations. The infant must learn about the permanence of objects that are temporarily obscured, the relation between retinal images, and the nearness of an object. He learns that by turning his head he will bring into view things that appeared at the edge of the field of vision, and that voices go with humans, and particular voices with particular humans.

The process of turning the brain into an instrument that can deal effectively with the myriad problems the world poses has been studied by developmental psychologists, the best-known probably being Jean Piaget. However, these theories will not be discussed here.

Anyone who has worked with minicomputers knows that when these devices are first switched on, there is very little one can do with them. The machinery is all there, the switches, the memory banks, the magnetic disks or tapes, and, most important, the central processor, which is the heart of the computer. But the system is unable to perform even the simplest calculation. It is necessary for the operator first to load into the computer memory a set of instructions known as the *bootstrap*. Only after it has absorbed the bootstrap can the machine perform the tasks for which it was designed. It can take data, store them, manipulate them in a great variety of ways, and it can learn different computer languages—that is, accept instructions in various ways that are convenient for the computer user.

Comparisons between brains and computers are often misleading, but the loading of the bootstrap is probably a good analogue to the transformations that take place in the maturing brain. In the case of the brain, however, it is often difficult to say how much is built-in design and how much the bootstrap of early experience.

How we see

Receiving and analyzing information about the world around us, and controlling our muscles to deal with it, are still the most engrossing functions of the human brain. We possess a *sensory-motor brain*. This expression reminds us that the chief task of all sensory input is to direct the body to carry out appropriate motor activities. This concept also aids in understanding the intricacies of sensory processing.

Since sight is the most highly developed of our senses, we will examine the mechanics and dynamics of seeing, and how, as we see, we act. We must keep in mind, however, that seeing is only one of the senses which act in concert to determine our actions. Another fact will soon emerge: Although sensing and doing are conceptually separable, they are functionally interlaced into a tight unit.

Close one eye, say your left one, and look out at a featureless background such as the ceiling or the sky. What you will see depends on the shape and size of your nose, but it will look something like a lopsided yin-yang diagram (Fig. 4.10). Look with the other eye, and you will see the mirror image. Look out with both eyes, and you will barely be aware of the obstacle in front of you. But your nose still blocks out part of the world from each eye and thus defines areas in the wings of the field of view which can be seen by one eye only. The rest of the panorama is under the simultaneous scrutiny of both eyes. We view the world *binocularly*, and this binocular vision gives us most of our sensation of depth, the three-dimensional quality of the visual scene.

Although all vertebrates have two eyes, not all are endowed with binocular vision. A parrot looks at you with its head cocked to the side, one eye facing you. The other, meanwhile, observes what is on the other side of its head. Very little is seen by both eyes at once.

I will now describe very briefly how visual information about the world is picked up by our eyes, and how this knowledge is handled and passed on through the successive populations of neurons that form the *visual pathway*.

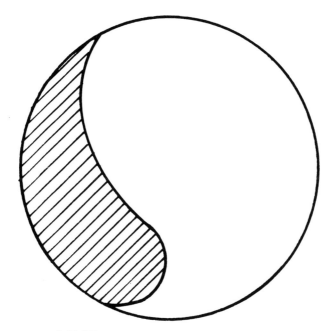

4.10 *The world seen with the right eye*

Rays of light enter each eye, the way light enters the lens of a camera. The lens of the eye focuses the rays on a surface behind the eye called the *retina*. All the visual features in front of us appear as a projected image on the retina, upside down, left and right interchanged, and much diminished in size. The impinging light falls on specialized cells called *photoreceptors,* which respond to the light with electrical signals.

There are two classes of photoreceptors in the vertebrate eye: the *rods* and the *cones*. They are distinguished by their shapes, from which their names are derived, and also by their different sensitivities to light intensities and to color. In the human eye about 100 million rods and cones are scattered over the retina like grains of photosensitive material in a photographic emulsion.

Besides the photoreceptors the retina contains a layer of neurons called *retinal ganglion cells* whose axons form the *optic nerve*. Between the photoreceptors and the ganglion cells is a network of different types of neurons that receives and passes on the electrical signals from the rods and cones. These neurons are the first stages of *visual information processing*. But first let us look at the position of the retina in the eye and the arrangement of cells within the retina.

Figure 4.11 shows a sketch of the human eye with lens, retina, and optic nerve, and a schematic drawing of the retina, greatly magnified, showing a network of cells intervening between receptors and ganglion cells. A curious fact emerges here: The rods and cones that constitute the photosensitive layer of the retina are on the *outside* surface of the retina, that is, the side facing away from the eyeball. The light that is focused here must first traverse several cell layers in the retina before reaching the photoreceptors. Similarly, the axons from the ganglion cells must cross the retina before emerging from the eye.

The intricacies of the retina are worth pondering for a moment. Visual information passes through distinct layers of cells, and what happens from one layer to the next can be considered a form of *mapping*. The pattern of light focused at the layer of photoreceptors is translated, or mapped, there into a pattern of electric potentials appearing as the outputs of the rods and cones. These signals are then picked up by the so-called *bipolar cells* (B in Fig. 4.11) and transmitted to the retinal ganglion cells. The *horizontal cells* (H) and the *amacrine cells* (A) convey signals *laterally* rather than straight through. These lateral interactions, which occur at all stages of sensory processing, show that more is involved here than simple, unmodified transmission of a pattern.

The retinal ganglion cells are the last level of processing in the retina. Their axons are bundled together into two large nerve cables, one for each eye: the *optic nerves*. There are roughly one million fibers in each optic nerve, corresponding to the one million retinal ganglion cells in each eye.

The two optic nerves proceed toward a part of the brain called the *thalamus*, where they terminate on two pieces of neural tissue, about the size of olives, called the *lateral geniculate nuclei* (LGN). But before reaching these structures, the fibers of the optic nerve undergo an important reordering in the big crossover of the *optic chiasm*. Here about half the fibers of each optic nerve cross to the other side of the brain.

It is important to mention that all senses, with the exception of the sense of smell, send their signals to specific locations in the thalamus. These *relay nuclei* then pass the information on to the neocortex.

In Fig. 4.12 I have drawn the principal features of the neural structures concerned with vision. The picture shows how an object appearing in front of us and to our right will be focused by the eye lenses on the left side of each retina; that is, on the outside, or *temporal*, side of

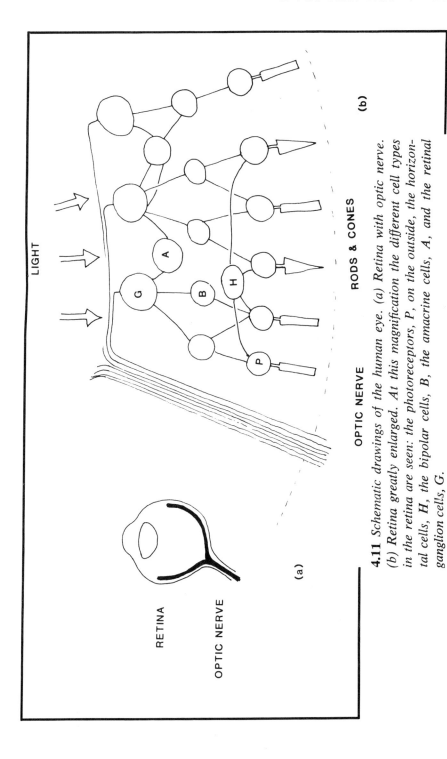

4.11 Schematic drawings of the human eye. (a) Retina with optic nerve. (b) Retina greatly enlarged. At this magnification the different cell types in the retina are seen: the photoreceptors, P, on the outside, the horizontal cells, H, the bipolar cells, B, the amacrine cells, A, and the retinal ganglion cells, G.

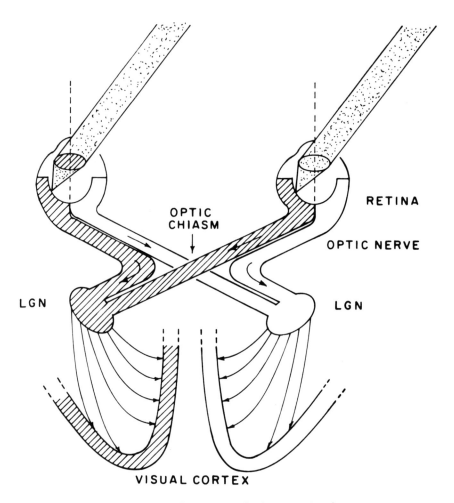

4.12 *Schematic drawing of the human visual system*

the left eye and on the *nasal* side of the right eye. In the rearrangement of the optic fibers at the chiasm, information from the temporal half of the left retina is routed to the left LGN. These fibers do not cross. They are joined there by the crossing fibers from the nasal half of the right eye.

Information about the object to our right is sent by *both* eyes to the left LGN. Similarly, the right LGN "sees" everything in the left half of the visual field through both eyes. The rearrangement of the fibers at the chiasm therefore has the following effect: Before the chiasm, each optic nerve carries *all* the information gathered by *one* eye. After the crossing, the optic nerve on one side reports only about the half of the world lying on the opposite side, but combines the information from both eyes.

From each LGN the nerve fibers (still about a million of them) radiate out and terminate in the neocortex on the same side. Thus the left cortex, just like the left LGN, "sees" the right half of the visual field through both eyes.

The visual process described above presents us with one of the major puzzles in vision. If you view a scene in front of you, the picture your brain receives is sharply divided down the middle, with the left and right portions going to opposite brain halves. And yet the scene is perceived as a whole, the matching of the two halves so perfect there is not a trace of a seam in the picture.

The axons coming from the retina terminate on successive layers of the LGN—there are six such layers in the human. From here, after only one synapse, the information goes to a place in the neocortex called the *visual cortex*.

We must now take a closer look at the LGN, because I believe that what happens here is crucial to our understanding of higher brain functions.

A layer of neurons in the LGN has some of the characteristics of the retina in that the position of each neuron in the layer corresponds to a similar position on the retina. This is another way of saying that if each active neuron in the LGN were to light up and if we could then *look* at the layer of neurons, we would find there a pattern of lights not very different from the pattern projected onto the retina by the lens, except that, of course, only one half of the retina is pictured. Because of this very graphic transformation of the retinal image into a pattern of activity in the LGN, the latter has been called an "internal retina."

On closer inspection we find two types of cells in the LGN: the *relay cells*, which receive signals from the retina and pass signals on to the cortex, and the *local circuit neurons*, or *interneurons*, which receive inputs from the retina as well as from relay cells but whose outputs affect only relay cells or other interneurons; that is, the axons of interneurons remain within the confines of the LGN. Figure 4.13 makes this distinction clear. The large circles on the left represent the one million retinal ganglion cells, and the large circles in the next layer to the right denote the relay cells in the LGN. The small circles are the interneurons in the LGN. Arrows represent excitatory synapses, dots indicate inhibitory synapses.

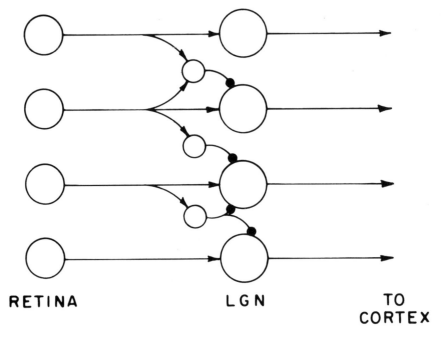

RETINA　　　　　　LGN　　　　　　TO
　　　　　　　　　　　　　　　　CORTEX

4.13 *Neural connections in one of the layers in the LGN*

Most of what we know about the functioning of this system comes
from studies in which minute electrodes are inserted into the brain to
pick up electrical signals from single neurons. In this way it is possible
to observe the responses of single cells in the retina, or the LGN, or
the cortex while different patterns of light are received by the eyes. We
would like to know what patterns of activity are created among the
millions of neurons in the visual pathway in response to a particular
scene. But experimental difficulties generally restrict us to the observation of just one neuron at a time. It is a common experimental technique, therefore, to vary the visual input and find out under what
conditions the rate of firing of a particular neuron is affected—either enhanced or depressed. The region in the visual field that must be illuminated for this to happen is called the *receptive field* of the cell. Figure
4.14 illustrates this point. A ganglion cell in the retina (G) receives
inputs from receptors lying within a narrow cone (E). Any light falling
on this part of the retina will increase the firing rate of this ganglion
cell. At the same time, (G) is less directly connected to receptors in
the larger cone (I). Light in this outer region tends to depress the ganglion cell's activity. We say that the *receptive field* of this cell consists

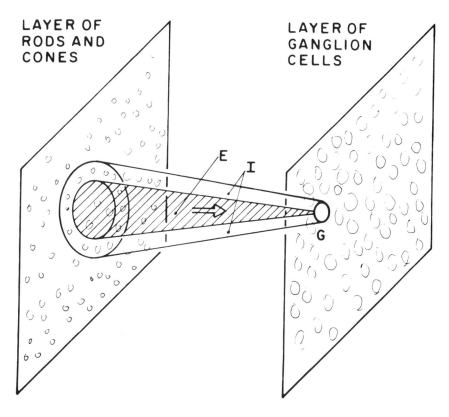

LAYER OF
RODS AND
CONES

LAYER OF
GANGLION
CELLS

4.14 *Receptive fields in the retina*

of an excitatory central region and an *inhibitory surround*. This is one
cell type but a very common one for ganglion cells.

Neighboring cells in the retina have neighboring and partially over-
lapping receptive fields. All retinal ganglion cells thus form a mosaic
of nearly circular fields covering all the visual field. The relay neurons
in the LGN form a similar mosaic and have similar responses.

Figure 4.14 also indicates that a ganglion cell in the retina may receive inputs from many receptors. This is especially true near the periphery of our field of vision. The number of rods and cones exceeds
the number of ganglion cells by a factor of about a hundred. Therefore,
there is a hundredfold *convergence* of paths from receptors to ganglion
cells. The mapping from ganglion cells to LGN, by contrast, is about
one-to-one.

We noted already that from each LGN about a million fibers radiate
out and carry information to the visual areas of the cortex. There is

one such area in each brain half, located in the extreme rear portion, the occipital pole of the brain. These visual areas consist of several sub-units (sometimes called visual areas I, II, and III) and involve several hundred million neurons. The million fibers from the LGN thus enter a system that is vast in comparison with the system in which they originated. This is an example of a strong *divergence* of pathways.

The techniques used to study activity in the visual cortex are the same as those applied to the more peripheral centers: recording the responses of single neurons contacted by a microelectrode. But, as one might expect, the behavior of these cells is more complicated and their function more obscure. The receptive fields no longer form simple mosaics of circular patches. David Hubel and Torsten Wiesel of Harvard University Medical School have discovered that cells in the visual cortex respond best to elongated patterns of light—lines or bars or edges of light, especially when they are flashed on suddenly or moved through the visual field.[13] A significant new feature appears here: The lines must be *oriented* at a particular angle—horizontal, vertical, or some intermediate angle—to produce a neural response. Each of the neurons examined was found to be *tuned* to a particular orientation. Other response characteristics were used by Hubel and Wiesel to classify these cells as *simple, complex,* and *hypercomplex.* Still, there appears to be a fair amount of order in this confusion. Cells with similar orientation preference are arranged in vertical "columns," and the angle of orientation changes smoothly as one traverses the cortex laterally.

What is the purpose of these receptive fields and their arrangement? A simpleminded interpretation is that these cells function as *detectors* of oriented lines, and that they are only the lowest members of a *hierarchy* of *feature detectors.* Somewhere higher up we might find cells tuned to particular familiar faces, the "grandmother neurons" of which we spoke in Chapter 3. There we also mentioned some of the conceptual difficulties that such a notion entails. There is also the suspicion among some physiologists that we have become overcommitted to interpreting visual phenomena in terms of the observed behavior of single neurons, and that our preoccupation with visual receptive fields may have led us into a conceptual cul-de-sac.

The visual cortex is by no means the last stage at which visual information appears in the brain. Although the difficulties of following the neural paths and the fate of the visual information beyond visual areas I, II, and III are staggering, a few general remarks can be made. In the large, relatively unexplored areas of the neocortex, neurons frequently respond to visual input, but almost never *exclusively* to such input. Most neurons in these so-called *association areas*, if they can be triggered at all, respond to a variety of sensory stimuli—visual, auditory, tactile, and others. Whether or not it makes sense to search for specific sensory phenomena to which these neurons may be tuned is still an open question. Such a search would at any rate be extremely difficult to carry out.

The supposition that there exists in the brain a hierarchy of feature-detecting cells seems to be losing ground. I argued earlier (see page 72) against what Francis Crick of DNA fame has recently called "the fallacy of the overwise neuron." Yet, features *are* detected by the brain, and the fact that such recognition in many cases leads to the execution of elaborate but predetermined action programs suggests that a simple and direct link must exist between the neurons involved in the detection and those responsible for action. We are led almost inevitably to a scheme like the one pictured in Fig. 3.1 (page 71), except that the link, the labeled command neuron, may be a population of neurons rather than a single cell.

Before talking about the motor side of this system, I want to mention a curious phenomenon called *blindsight*. It was observed that monkeys which had had the visual cortex completely removed were nevertheless able to solve some visual discrimination tasks and avoid obstacles in locomotion. The explanation for this surprising fact is found in the existence of two visual systems, only one of which is shown in Fig. 4.12. Not shown is a part of the optic nerve which branches off between the retina and the LGN and leads directly to a place in the midbrain, and from there via part of the thalamus to the neocortex. It is believed that the residual vision observed in monkeys without their visual cortex is due to this "second visual system."

The phenomenon has now been observed in humans also. It was known for some time that a person who is blind over a certain portion of his visual field may nevertheless move his eyes in response to a flash of light appearing in the insensitive region. The common explanation is again that the *second visual system*, which in man controls eye movements, is unimpaired and can guide the eyes toward a source of light that is not consciously *seen*.

In a more recent experiment, L. Weiskrantz and his collaborators at the National Hospital in Queen Square, London, set out to investigate whether other visual faculties may exist in blind regions of the visual field. They reported one case of a patient who had lost vision over one half of his visual field due to the surgical removal of most of the visual cortex on one side.[14] Such a defect is called *hemianopia*. A person with this problem sees with both eyes, but the world in front of him is neatly cut off on one side of a vertical line through the center of his gaze. If a person with hemianopia fixes his gaze on a point on a screen, and if an experimenter flashes spots of light at various locations on that screen, the person will be aware of the stimuli only when the flashes occur on one side of the point of fixation, the normal *hemifield*. Weiskrantz's patient, having lost his right visual cortex, had a normal hemifield on the right and was blind in the left hemifield. Into this blind region Weiskrantz projected light in patterns of X's and O's in random order. As expected, the subject, when asked, stated that he saw nothing. When urged to make a choice, however, he guessed correctly in twenty-seven out of thirty trials. In another run the choice was between horizontal and vertical stripes. This time he was correct thirty times in thirty trials. The patient continued to maintain that he was unaware of seeing *anything* and showed surprise when informed of his success rate.

The most likely explanation for these results is probably the same as before: Visual information is conducted from the eyes to a place in the midbrain, thus bypassing the defective visual cortex. This second visual system not only serves to direct our gaze at moving targets but is capable of performing discriminatory tasks. What makes this phenomenon so remarkable, however, is that in addition to the existence of a visual backup system it is also possible to receive useful sensory information without being conscious of it. Consciousness appears here for the first time not as a necessary concomitant of sensory signals received but as something additional, a sensory extravaganza we could perhaps do without.

Finally, to complicate matters further, Tore Torjussen of the University of Oslo, Norway, reported three cases of *conscious* blindsight.[15] His subjects, like Weiskrantz's patient, suffered from hemianopia due to different brain pathologies. Visual patterns were presented and the subjects asked to describe what they saw. Torjussen used an ingenious technique to avoid two sources of confusion that plague experiments of this sort. It is important to prevent a shift in the subject's gaze, so that one can be sure which portion of the stimulus is in the normal and which in the blind region of the field. This is sometimes achieved by using a device called a *tachistoscope,* which flashes the pattern on for a brief instant. This prevents any shift in the point of fixation during the viewing and forces the subject to describe what he saw "from memory." It is possible that the imagination of the viewer may play a significant role in his reported reaction. Torjussen wanted a report on what the subject saw, not what he thought he had seen. He used a flash that lasted for only one thousandth of a second, but it was of such intensity that the subject was able to view an afterimage against a blank background. The intensity of the background illumination changed abruptly from bright to dark, which further enhanced the quality and duration of the afterimage. Any movement of the eyes while observing the afterimage moved the afterimage itself, so the position of the point of fixation relative to the image remained fixed.

Torjussen describes the responses to various visual stimuli, some of which were entirely in the normal half of the field, some in the hemianopic field, and some that straddled the two hemifields. The patterns are drawn in the upper four diagrams (S1–S4) of Fig. 4.15. The crosses mark the points of fixation of the subjects. Here S1 is a complete circle straddling the vertical midline; the right half entirely in the blind hemifield is shown as a shaded area. The second stimulus is a half-circle lying entirely in the normal field. Diagram S3 is a half-circle entirely in the hemianopic field, and S4 represents two half-circles displaced with respect to each other and straddling the midline as shown.

Below these stimulus patterns are the patterns reported "seen" by the subjects. The complete disk, S1, produced the sensation of a complete disk, even though half of it was in the blind hemifield. But the half disk, S2, in the normal field was perceived as what it is: a half-disk. Apparently light falling into the blind area *does* make a difference in the conscious sensation. But showing the half-disk, S3, alone in the blind field produced no conscious sensation. Torjussen concluded that to "see" something in the blind region, there must be a stimulus in the blind hemifield as well as in the symmetrically located portion of the normal field. This supposition is confirmed in a startling way by the responses to stimulus S4. Besides the half-disk on the left, the subjects *saw* that portion of the illuminated blind area which was also symmetrical with the pattern appearing in the normal hemifield.

These experiments are relatively new and involve only a few subjects. If we tried to generalize from them, and this is admittedly speculative, we would deduce that humans are able to discriminate light patterns in the hemianopic portions of their visual field, but that *conscious* sensation is lacking unless the illuminated area in the blind

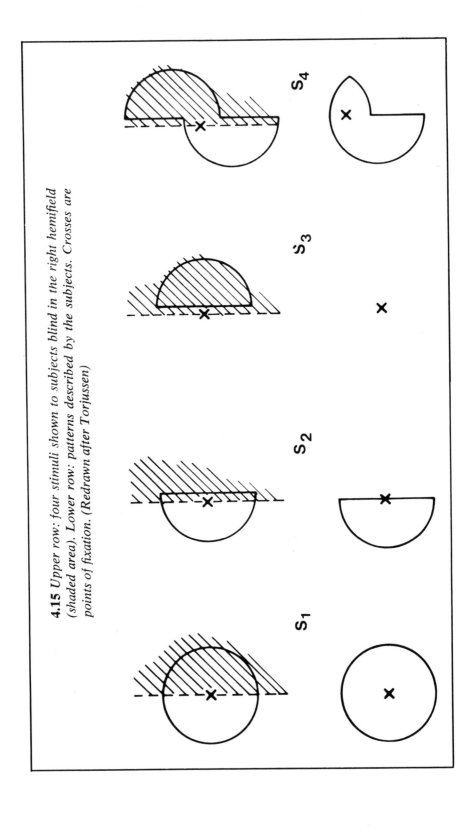

4.15 Upper row: four stimuli shown to subjects blind in the right hemifield (shaded area). Lower row: patterns described by the subjects. Crosses are points of fixation. (Redrawn after Torjussen)

region is contiguous to and symmetrical with a pattern in the normal hemifield.

The diagram of the visual pathway sketched in Fig. 4.12 is incomplete in another important respect. The LGN is not just a simple relay station carrying messages from retina to cortex but receives inputs from at least two other regions. One region is the *reticular activating system* (RAS) mentioned earlier on page 99 as the system that arouses the cortex into consciousness. It appears to have a similar *gating* effect on the LGN. The other input comes from the cortex itself. These connections run counter to the main stream of visual information and are called *corticofugal* fibers, mentioned earlier on page 102. These fibers appear to originate in different parts of the cortex and make a variety of synapses with cells in the LGN. They are evidently able to modify the ability of LGN relay neurons to pass on their sensory information.

Again, the visual system described here in some detail is a prototype for the other senses. We mentioned that, with one exception, all afferent sensory pathways go through relay nuclei in the thalamus. It is probably true also that all these sensory nuclei receive strong inputs from corticofugal fibers as well as from the RAS.

There have been many conjectures about the function of these pathways. It is clear that some modulating influence is exerted by the cortex on the entering sensory signals. One particular example of such cortical selection has recently emerged. The images from the two eyes, brought together in the LGN, interact there through mutually inhibitory connections. This well-known phenomenon causes *ocular competition* and generally makes one eye dominate over the other. It was found that the cortex will *override* that competition for points in the visual field lying in the plane of fixation. This means that when we view an object, the two retinal images which are *in register* will be transmitted equally to the cortex, while for nearer or farther objects, one of the disparate views will be suppressed. This selection and important modification of what we see is accomplished by the corticofugal connections to the LGN.

The relationship between the different components of the visual system is shown in Fig. 4.16 and can now be summarized as follows: Visual patterns are first projected by the lens system of the eye onto the surface of the photoreceptors. The resulting electrical activity is propagated through several layers of cells in the retina. The information then emerges through the fibers of the optic nerve as a pattern of action potentials. After the reordering of fibers in the chiasm, the optic

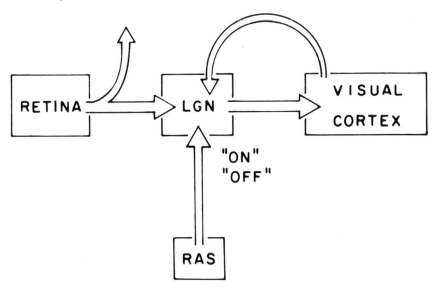

4.16 *Information flow through the visual system (retina-LGN-visual cortex), showing the switching action of the RAS and feedback control of the LGN by the cortex.*

nerve terminates on the LGN, a structure of several cell layers, each of which reproduces the pattern of activity sent by the retina. Before reaching the LGN, a part of the optic nerve branches off from the main trunk and heads for a place in the midbrain. This is the beginning of what has been called the "second visual system."

Going back to the main branch, the LGN sends its signals to visual areas I, II, and III in the cerebral cortex. We did not attempt to follow the information farther into the depths of the cortex. We did, however, stress one aspect that both complicates and enriches the picture immeasurably: The LGN is more than a simple relay. This "internal retina" can be turned on and off as effectively as we blink our eyes. This is accomplished by fibers coming from the RAS. In addition, the cortex can modify the activity at the LGN through its corticofugal fibers and thereby manipulate its own input. Chapter 5 will discuss further this remarkable aspect of sensory processing.

The above sketch of the structure and function of the human visual system is incomplete. Still, to the uninitiated reader this may all have seemed quite involved and perhaps a bit tedious. We said almost nothing about stereo vision, nothing at all about the chemical processes that translate light stimuli into electrical signals in the rods and cones, or anything about the nature of color vision or the perception of motion—all important elements in vision. However, excellent sources are available that describe these topics and I will excuse my shortcomings with the remark of a wise teacher who once said that instead of covering everything it is better to uncover a little.

In the next section we will make the transition from the sensory to the motor side of the brain, and we will find there is a fuzzy boundary

How we do

We have used the expression *sensory-motor brain*. In general, motor activity is the ultimate purpose of all brain function. It would be of no use to the animal to sense and recognize its predators if it were not able also to effect an escape.

But not all perception leads to action. Consider a person looking at a shop window. There is a continuous stream of visual information entering the nervous system: Merchandise of all types is scanned, and prices are noted. But, apart from the occasional shifting of the gaze, little overt action results from all this information until after a while the person walks away.

When action occurs this happens, as a rule, at the end of a chain of events that begins at the sense receptors, progresses through stages called *information-processing*, and ends with the triggering of effector neurons and the contracting of muscles. This causal chain is a good way to begin our study of action, though we will find it an inadequate explanation in many instances.

First of all, there are the motor functions that require neither an external sensory trigger nor an act of volition. The actions of the heart and lungs, and the *visceral functions* belong in that category. The appropriate muscles are controlled by the *autonomic nervous system*, which keeps functioning like a superb machine for our entire life-span whether we are awake or asleep. We will talk in this section about the *voluntary muscles*. Most of these are involved with the motion of our limbs, and are called the *skeletal muscles*.

Consider the following two situations. In the first you are standing at a podium, addressing a crowd, when suddenly someone throws something at you. You react quickly by ducking, thus avoiding the missile. The causal chain stands out clearly here: the visual input, recognized by your nervous system as an object heading in your direction, the interpretation of the event as potentially dangerous or unpleasant, and the motor commands to take evasive action. The entire sequence is over in less than a second.

The other situation is quite different. A man stands on a bridge looking motionlessly at the waters far below him. Suddenly, he vaults over the railing—to his death.

I pick a particularly dramatic example to make a point: This last action was not caused by an immediate sensory trigger. What led up to the tragic act all took place within the nervous system. "An act like this," says Albert Camus, "is prepared within the silence of the heart, as is a great work of art."

Work of art or not, the action described here, and many others of a less tragic nature, are the result of lengthy "mental" activity that can extend over minutes or years, and whose detailed dynamics cannot easily be reconstructed.

We distinguish three modes of operation of the brain. In the first mode (the window shopper) sensations are received but do not elicit overt action. These inputs may go virtually unnoticed, or may lead to lively mental activity involving recognition, storing of information, wonder, curiosity, and, in the case of the shopper, perhaps dismay. In the second mode ((b) in Fig. 4.17) sensory input leads quickly to

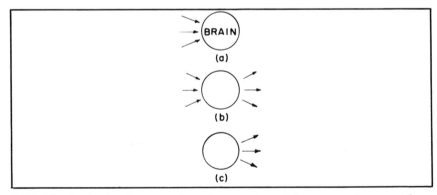

4.17 *The brain in three modes of operation: (a) sensory input without action; (b) action triggered sensory input; (c) action without sensory trigger*

motor output (ducking a thrown object), while in the third mode (the suicide, or (c) in Fig. 4.17) motor action appears spontaneously, even capriciously.

Since this section is concerned with action, we are interested in the last two cases. As with most classifications, the distinction is somewhat arbitrary and oversimplified. Generalizing a little further, it can be said that case two (b) would properly be studied by a physiologist, while case three (c) might be analyzed by a behavioral psychologist or a psychiatrist. No theory of brain function, however, is complete that does not take into account the cases shown as diagrams (a) and (c) in Fig. 4.17, in which the flow of information is *not* a smooth and rapid progression from receptors to effectors. It is precisely when this simple hierarchy breaks down that we are faced with what are often called the "higher brain functions."

This is not to say that the sensory-motor causal chain is simple. Many brain centers are involved in the performance of even the most rudimentary tasks, and their interactions pose formidable questions. The Swedish neurophysiologist and Nobel laureate Ragnar Granit, in a particularly pessimistic mood, stated that "scientists may have to abandon the hope of ever understanding the whole miraculous performance of our sensory-motor brain."[16]

This section will outline the function of some of the components of these efferent pathways. In Chapter 5 we will come back to the even more challenging situations depicted by diagrams (a) and (c) in Fig. 4.17.

We will begin this discussion at the end of the chain—at the muscles. These consist of cells which, like the neurons, have excitable membranes. When certain *transmitter molecules* are present, the muscle fiber contracts. The transmitter is a substance called *acetylcholine,* which is secreted at synapses at the end of the axon of a *motoneuron.* The place where the transmission from neuron to muscle occurs is called a *neuromuscular junction.* This is a synapse, much like the one shown in Fig. 2.11 (page 53) except that the axon terminates on a muscle fiber instead of on the dendrite of another neuron. Figure 4.18 shows an incoming axon with its terminal *end plate* making a synapse on a muscle fiber.

The American Indians used a much dreaded poison, *curare,* on their arrows to paralyze their enemies. We know now that this drug (used in modern medicine) prevents the transmission of acetylcholine

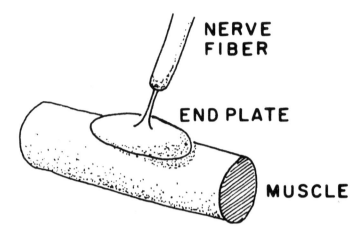

NERVE
FIBER

END PLATE

MUSCLE

4.18 *Axon from a motoneuron terminating on a section of muscle fiber, making a typical* neuromuscular junction

between the nerve end plate and the muscle fiber. Thus the action commands from the brain reach the motoneurons but never get to the muscles. Humans given curare for medicinal reasons are conscious and have thoughts but can neither speak nor gesture. The sensations accompanying paralysis by curare have recently been described most lucidly by John Stevens, a physiologist at the School of Medicine of the University of Pennsylvania. Stevens himself was the subject of an experiment in which certain ideas concerning consciousness in motor control were tested. Stevens reports:

> I was the subject for those total paralysis experiments and can assure anyone who wishes to repeat them that the major perceptions were quite unambiguous—one felt like a solid piece of cement. It was very much like being buried alive. Not only was voluntary movement impossible, but one was painfully aware that it was impossible. There was never any phantom perception of either limb movement or limb position. The perception of paralysis or immobility was just as dramatic for the extraocular muscles. Any attempt to move the eyes left or right was met with a sense of stark immobility.[17]

The motoneurons are located in the spinal cord, where populations, or *pools*, of such cells are found together with interneurons, coupled to one another by excitatory and inhibitory synapses and sending axons to the various muscles.

The skeletal muscles, which move our limbs, are made to contract by the action of motoneurons in the spinal cord. These are called *alpha* motoneurons. The links between these cells and muscle fibers are the neuromuscular junctions mentioned on page 135. The muscles in turn contain *sensors,* which report the accomplished action back to the spinal cord. The sensors are part of the so-called *muscle spindles* and belong to a system of sensory apparatus whose function it is to inform the central nervous system of the status of our limb positions. This is called the *proprioceptive system.*

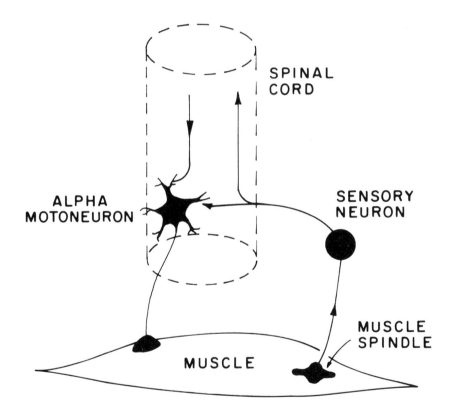

4.19 *Nervous control of a skeletal muscle and sensory response*

Figure 4.19 shows an alpha motoneuron in the spinal cord with its efferent fiber going to a skeletal muscle. From the muscle spindle, which is stretched or squeezed as the muscle moves, axons convey messages back to the spinal cord. Note also that this sensory information is sent up the cord to the brain. Similarly, the alpha motoneurons may receive their instructions from the brain. Figure 4.19 also shows that the muscle-spindle sensors send axon branches to alpha motoneurons.

We are now in a position to follow the dynamics of an important neuromuscular function: the *stretch reflex*. It begins when one of the skeletal muscles is stretched by some external means. This will also elongate the muscle spindle and cause the sensors to send impulses back to the spinal cord. There these signals are able to trigger alpha motoneurons. These in turn, by activating neuromuscular junctions, cause the skeletal muscle to contract. The effect of the stretch reflex, in sum, is that a muscle that is forcibly elongated responds with a contraction.

The knee jerk is the best-known example of a stretch reflex. The muscle involved is the extensor of the lower leg. Stretching the muscle is accomplished by hitting the tendon to which it is attached just below the kneecap. The response is immediate and cannot be prevented by voluntary commands from the brain. This is only the simplest example of many motor functions that are controlled by neural circuits within the spinal cord.

The motor system contains one other very significant complication. Within the muscle spindle, which is embedded in a skeletal muscle, are the so-called *intrafusal muscles*. These are arranged at either end of the sensory element of the spindle in such a way that they pull on the sensor and cause it to fire whenever they contract (Fig. 4.20). These intrafusal muscles are also triggered by neuromuscular junctions. The neural fibers responsible for this are called *gamma* fibers and come from *gamma motoneurons* in the spinal cord. I want to stress that the contraction of the intrafusal muscles only affects the sensors in the muscle spindle, but does not produce any body motion directly.

Consider now the effect of the gamma motoneurons. These cells are also in the spinal cord. Their axons make neuromuscular junctions with the intrafusal muscle fibers. When gamma motoneurons fire, intrafusal muscles contract. But since the skeletal muscle fiber has not moved, this will again stretch the muscle spindle and cause it to fire, triggering the alpha motoneuron and causing the muscle to contract. In general, activity in the gamma motoneuron has the same effect as stretching the muscle. Therefore, the activity of the muscle spindle will depend on both the elongation of the muscle and on the activity of the gamma motoneuron.

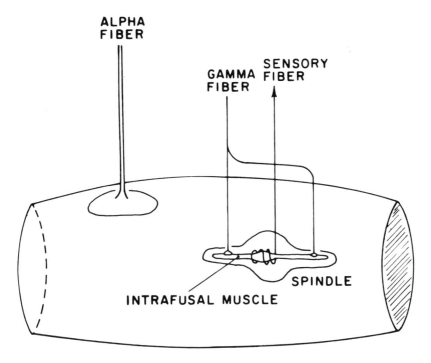

SKELETAL MUSCLE

4.20 *The muscle spindle*

The intrafusal muscles add a new dimension to the picture of motor control and motor sensation. We have here another example of how the central nervous system reaches out to the periphery to manipulate its own sensory input, since it controls the gamma motoneurons, which alter the response of muscle receptors to true, or skeletal, motion.

The preceding discussion included only some of the simplest connections in the spinal cord and some of the most primitive functions. The interactions between the various types of motoneurons, the muscle spindles, and other sensors that report back to the spinal cord, as well as the interneurons that exist there in large numbers, give rise to a great variety of *spinal reflexes* of which the knee jerk is one of the most primitive. Much more complex motor functions, such as scratching or even walking, are fully programmed spinal reflexes and can be carried out, if somewhat clumsily, by mammals without any help from the brain.

Many of the motor functions of which the spinal cord is capable can also be done *voluntarily*, that is, under control from the brain. Such control comes primarily from a part of the cortex called the *motor cortex*. This structure lies in a strip just forward of a prominent fissure, the *central sulcus*, which runs laterally across the center of the cerebral hemispheres (Fig. 4.21).

In the motor area of the cortex we find a particularly large type of neuron, the *Betz cell*. The axons of these neurons form a large *descending* tract—about one million fibers in humans—the *pyramidal tract*. Most of these fibers enter the spinal cord, where they make synapses on interneurons or directly on motoneurons. This is one of the sources of the brain's control of motor functions.

Here then is the chain of command: from the Betz cells in the motor cortex to the motoneurons (both alpha and gamma) in the spinal cord, and from there to the muscles. At the uppermost part of this chain, in the motor cortex, we are once again in the rarefied regions of the highest brain functions, and within whispering distance of that part of the cortex that *receives* all sorts of sensory input concerning body position and body movement: the *somatosensory cortex*. The place where the motor cortex abuts the somatosensory cortex, at the bottom of the central sulcus, corresponds to the hyphen in the expression "sensory-motor brain." It is a unique part of the cortex and perhaps the most crucial.

We have discussed one type of muscle receptor, the muscle spindle, and how it reports back to the spinal cord. From there the sensory fibers continue on to the cortex.

The muscle spindle is only one of a number of sense organs that watch over body position and motion. Others are the *tendon organs,* which measure tension in the muscle tendons, and receptors located in the skeletal joints, the *joint receptors*. Supplemental information comes from different sense organs located in the skin (*cutaneous senses*), from the sense of balance (*vestibular system*) located in the inner ear, and, of course, from vision. All these sense data find their way to the somatosensory cortex. There, gathered from many sources, is the complete picture of our body's disposition in space and its motions.

We now perceive a giant loop that spans the entire breadth and depth of brain function: from the motor cortex down the pyramidal tract and spinal cord to the skeletal muscles; and from the sensors in the muscles, joints, and skin, as well as the senses of balance and vision, all the way back to the somatosensory cortex, right next to the

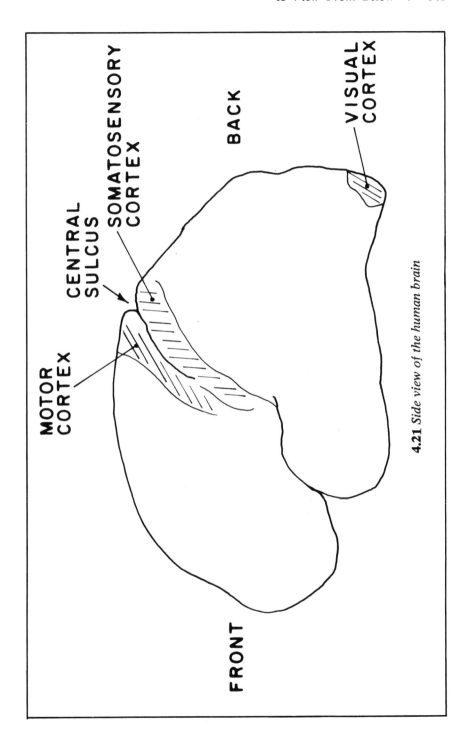

MOTOR CORTEX

CENTRAL SULCUS

SOMATOSENSORY CORTEX

BACK

VISUAL CORTEX

FRONT

4.21 *Side view of the human brain*

motor cortex from which we started out (Fig. 4.22). The side branches and smaller loops—to the cerebellum, the brainstem, the thalamus—are also important, but a consideration of these would take us too far afield.

Both the motor and somatosensory cortices can readily be subdivided according to the different parts of the body they represent. Pictures are frequently drawn in which a human figure, with its parts quite distinct if somewhat distorted, is laid out along each of the two parallel strips of cortex on either side of the central sulcus. As might be expected, a sensitive and delicately controllable part such as the human hand occupies a disproportionately large area. The same is true for the head, particularly the lips and tongue. By comparison, the space allotted to the legs is relatively small. It is significant to note that as we cross the central sulcus from the sensory to the motor cortex, the body part represented remains generally the same: the sensory and motor images of the thumb, for example, directly oppose each other across the central sulcus.

So much for structure. As soon as we begin to ask about the *functioning* of the motor system, we are faced with a number of fundamental questions. How are the cortical motor commands formulated when they are triggered by a sensory event? What forms the commands when the action is voluntary and spontaneous? How are ongoing activities, such as steering an automobile or guiding a paint brush, observed and checked for their desired effect, and how is the motor system directed to make appropriate corrections? To what extent does the cortex anticipate a whole sequence of events and lay out in advance a sequence of motor actions? Is it possible that all corrections are made *subcortically*—for example, in the spinal cord—by checking for deviations from the original master plan?

On the last question, the consensus among physiologists seems to be now that continuous progress reports from the various senses reach the cortex, where they are able to cause the revision of ongoing programs. How this feedback control works is by no means clear, but I will venture some guesses in Chapter 5. The chief difficulty is that the supposed comparison involves two quite dissimilar things, like apples and oranges. One is a set of motor commands directing specific motoneurons to fire, the other a mixture of different sensory reports on muscle tension, limb position, and motion. Also the corresponding neural activities appear in adjacent but distinct cortical areas—the motor cortex and the somatosensory cortex.

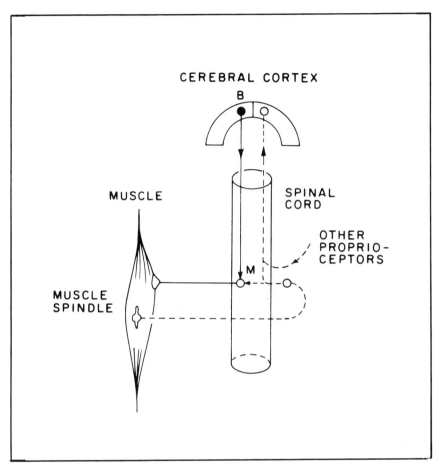

4.22 *The great sensory-motor loop. Efferent paths from a Betz cell, B, in the motor cortex via the pyramidal tract to the motoneuron, M, in the spinal cord, to the muscle. Sensory pathways (dotted lines) from the muscle spindle, tendon organs, and other senses to the somatosensory cortex.*

According to another prevalent theory, the motor commands issuing from the cortex are copied somewhere on the way out and kept as a reference against which performance can be checked. This is sometimes called a *feed-forward* scheme, and the saved motor program is called an *efference copy*. There is, however, no direct evidence that such a copy is ever made, and no clue as to where in the brain it might be stored. Again, any comparison between efference copy and sensory reports runs into this fundamental difficulty: They are expressed in different languages.

In answer to the other questions raised above, we must equally admit our ignorance. In such fast, triggered actions as ducking a missile or recovering equilibrium after stumbling over an unseen object, our knowledge of the linkage between receptors and effectors is highly incomplete, with only here and there the beginning of a true understanding. As we have pointed out repeatedly, the processes must include, on the sensory side of the brain, mechanisms for the detection and recognition of *features*, and, on the motor side, readily available *motorprograms*. Most important, circuitry must exist that connects the recognition of specific features with the activation of appropriate action programs.

The spontaneous generation of voluntary action is an even more elusive process. In this case, concrete commands emerge unpredictably out of the nebulous realm of thought processes. Recent experiments on voluntary motion have produced some interesting and surprising results, to be discussed in Chapter 5, which is devoted to the *mind*.

Pain!

Of all sensations pain is the one most clearly linked to consciousness. We can be "deliriously happy," "peacefully asleep," but pain is quintessential awareness. Numerous colloquialisms in the English language recognize this consciousness-rallying quality of pain. The opposite of being blissfully unaware is to be *painfully aware* of something. Of course, we can be conscious of pleasure, but painful unawareness is a contradiction in terms. Pain is at the beginning of life and, for most of us, the last sensation.

Unlike most sensations, pain has a compelling quality. It urges us irresistibly to protect our bodies from harm, to nurse our injuries and ills, to preserve our lives. But pain in its extreme form, *chronic pain,* can also be devastating, making life itself unbearable. Such pain was characterized by Walle Nauta of MIT as constituting "a change in the whole internal set of the organism, an existential state rather than a sensory one."[18]

What is it that makes pain unique among the senses? We can enumerate a few distinctions, but they hardly account for the almost mysterious quality of the phenomenon.

In the sensations of sight, sound, touch, and others, we can usually point to physical entities that are the sources of the sensations, and to qualities of the sources that are described by the sensations. The sound of a bell is *projected* (see pages 99–100) by the brain to the bell tower, and its timbre is heard as a *quality of the bell*. Similarly, when I look at the sky my sensation of blueness, although subjective, is nevertheless experienced as a *quality of the sky*, just as heat or cold are felt as qualities of objects being touched.

This *projection* ceases abruptly, however, the moment the sensation becomes one of pain. The pain I feel when I burn myself on a stovetop is *not* a quality of the stovetop. The stove, in fact, has suddenly become irrelevant. My attention is instead riveted on *my pain. It* is the *thing* that is being sensed. Such objectification is characteristic of pain. It *resides* in a particular part of the body. Sometimes it *comes and goes*, but it is an object that is peculiarly *mine*. It cannot be sampled by anyone else, and it has no existence without me. The characteristic feature of pain is not projection but retrenchment.

It is not difficult to see the purpose of this shift of attention from object to self. The sound of a bell tells me something interesting about the bell, but the scream of a siren close to my ears has a much more urgent message: Protect my ears before they are irreparably damaged. Thus pain signifies damage, or the danger of damage to tissue from external or internal sources. But what is the neural basis for this urgency, this irresistibility? Suppose I really don't care about the damage. Why can't I just take note of the warning—and calmly ignore it? This is a quality of pain sensation that is still least understood.

In many other respects, pain is not unlike other senses. It has receptors that are distributed through the body; it has neural pathways leading to the brain, most of them going through the spinal cord; and, of course, it has *loops*. We will now take a look at this neural circuitry, as much of it as is known.

The best-known pain pathways originate at the surface of the body —the skin. Located here are a number of senses, the *cutaneous senses*, among them pressure, temperature (actually separate senses for heat and cold), and pain.

There has been a long-standing dispute whether the receptors and the fibers carrying pain messages from the skin are the same as those of temperature and perhaps touch, or whether there are pathways specializing in pain. There are three theories in this regard. According to the theory of *intensity coding,* any of the skin senses, in fact any sense at all, will produce a sensation of pain when overstimulated. An overdriven touch or temperature receptor will elicit pain, as will the receptors in the retina when light becomes too intense. In this theory there are no specialized pain receptors.

According to another theory, pain is not so much the result of excessive firing in single fibers, but is due to a particular *pattern* of activity among populations of afferent fibers. As in intensity coding, the *pattern theory* has no receptors dedicated solely to the transmission of pain information.

Finally, in the *specificity theory* some receptors fire only when stimulation exceeds the pain threshold. They and their associated afferent fibers form a neural system exclusively dedicated to pain.

The issues are by no means completely resolved, but the specificity theory is currently favored by most physiologists. Two types of nerve fibers are now believed to be responsible for pain conduction: the moderately fast "A-delta fibers" and the system of very small, slowly conducting "C-fibers." The sensory endings of these nerves are distributed throughout the skin. However, not all of these are pain receptors. Some respond to temperature or to various forms of mechanical stimulation.

The two pain *channels* are not only different in their speed of conduction but they also carry different *qualities* of pain. The sensation conveyed by the faster A-delta channel is of a sharp, localized pain. C-fiber pain is dull, aching or burning, and poorly localized. It is also deep and lasting, and sometimes reaches intolerable intensities.

It is not clear how the sensory endings of the cutaneous pain receptors are stimulated. Tissue damage by excessive heat or pressure, or tissue disruption, releases a number of chemicals, among them serotonin, histamine, and *bradykinin*. Some pain receptors are particularly sensitive to one or another of these, and it has been conjectured that the triggering of these nerve endings is always through some specific chemical. It was found, for example, that fluid extracted from injured tissue caused pain when injected at an uninjured site. This gives support to the idea of chemical stimulation.

There may also be a special transmitter substance operating in the neural pathways that convey pain sensation. This is a chemical belonging to a class called *neuropeptides* and has been given the name *substance P*.

Tolerance of pain and behavioral responses vary greatly from individual to individual. However, there is remarkable agreement when different people are asked whether or not a particular stimulus is painful. Such experiments can be carried out readily by controlling skin temperature. Most subjects will call a temperature in excess of about 45 degrees centigrade (113 degrees Fahrenheit) painful. This is also the temperature at which tissue damage begins to occur.

As in the case of vision, we can follow the sensory pathways of pain from the receptors "upward" to different parts of the brain, but details of the connections are poorly known. As stated, two main pathways can be distinguished. One conducts the fast A-delta information on sharp pain through the spinal cord to specific relay nuclei in the thalamus, and from there to the somatosensory cortex. (This is analogous to the main visual pathway from the retina to the lateral geniculate nucleus (LGN) to the visual cortex, as discussed on pages 120–123.) The other tract, carrying mostly the slower C-fibers, goes through the spinal cord and terminates in the *reticular activating system* (RAS), a structure that extends upward from the brainstem and into the thalamus. The two tracts are shown schematically in Fig. 4.23.

On pages 99 and 131 we noted that the RAS has the interesting function of *arousing* the cerebral cortex, which without RAS input would be permanently comatose. Through the RAS the C-fibers exert a powerful alerting action on all parts of the cortex. The excitement, the urgency that go with severe pain are probably the result of the diffuse and highly complex influence the RAS has on the rest of the brain.

As in the case of the visual system, the pain pathways do not carry just one-way traffic from the sensors to the brain. Here, too, there is evidence of strong feedback "from above." *Corticofugal control* is exerted on all intermediate stations, all the way down to the spinal cord. (I have not shown these descending paths in Fig. 4.23 in order to keep the diagram simple.)

When an injury occurs somewhere on the surface of the body, pain is usually not the only sensation telling us that something has happened. We often see or hear the cause of the injury. We can also inspect the damage visually or through touch. But, most important, we know—again mostly by sight or by touch—what the normal state of affairs should be. But not in the case of internal, or *visceral*, pain. To say, "I have a pain in the stomach" or "the left kidney" is truly an *educated* guess, since the brain has no firsthand knowledge that there is such a thing as a stomach or a kidney. It is not that the interior of the body lacks sensors. There are many senses (the so-called *enteroceptors*) which continually check on the internal milieu and control muscular and glandular functions vital to our continual well-being.

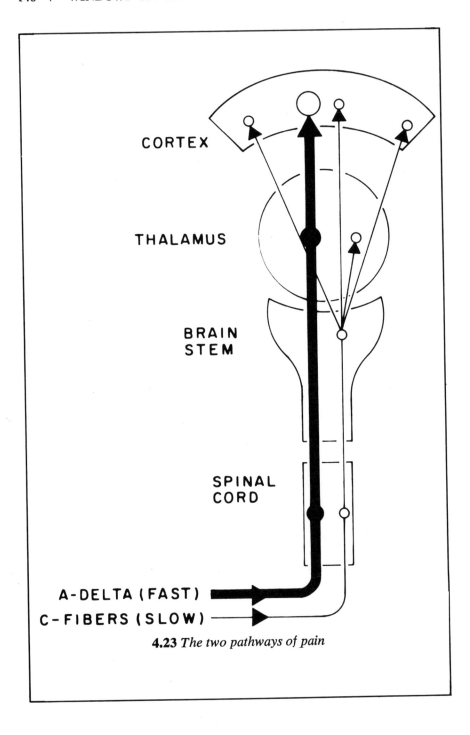

CORTEX

THALAMUS

BRAIN
STEM

SPINAL
CORD

A-DELTA (FAST)
C-FIBERS (SLOW)

4.23 *The two pathways of pain*

However, most of these control, or *homoeostatic,* functions are not consciously perceived.

Visceral pain often does not even seem to come from the affected organ, but is *referred* instead to some location on the surface of the body. Some best-known examples are the referred pains of cardiac ischemia (insufficient blood supply to the heart muscle) which seem to originate at the base of the neck, the shoulders, and the upper arms.

We know much less about the pathways of visceral pain reception than about cutaneous pain. However, the fibers involved are A-delta and C-fiber types, and join the cutaneous fibers in the two main tracts that lead up the spinal cord to the brain. Bradykinin, the painful chemical we encountered in the skin, again seems to be involved in visceral and muscle pain.

Pain can be modified by a number of factors, most of them poorly understood. Stimulating the fast-conducting surface senses of pressure or temperature often reduces a painful sensation. Rubbing the skin near a painful location has that effect. This is often explained as resulting from a mutually inhibitory interaction between the fast and slow fiber systems in the spinal cord. There is some speculation that *gates* exist in the spinal cord whereby pain inputs can be shut off there before they reach the brain. Rubs with ointments that produce lasting skin stimulation and reduce pain in deep tissue such as joints and muscles probably work on this principle.

Pain inhibition can be achieved also by electrical stimulation of parts of the cerebral cortex or the thalamus, which may act via descending fibers on the same spinal gates and block the incoming pain signals. Neurosurgery has helped in some but not all cases of otherwise intractable pain.

This brings up the question of where in the nervous system the ultimate sensation of pain takes place. This is as elusive as the location of memory. Lesions in the thalamus were found to block chronic pain but not acute pain. It is reported that even complete removal of the cerebral cortex does not necessarily abolish all pain. On the other hand, pain can be produced by some lesions in the cortex. Surface pain often persists after the afferent tracts of pain-conducting fibers have been cut. The *phantom limb* is a well-known phenomenon in which pain sensations can persist in parts long severed from the body. Many amputees suffer from this phenomenon.

Where, then, *is* pain? Its true neurological basis is still obscure. There are also emotional components that affect our sensations in mysterious ways. We apparently can be talked into or talked out of having pain, if we believe the claims about hypnosis. We don't know whether acupuncture works through physical or psychological mechanisms, or whether it even makes sense to distinguish between the two.

The emotional components of pain are also its most devastating aspects. Fear, anguish, despair all add to pain's misery, but seem to have different locations and involve different mechanisms. Patients who have undergone frontal lobotomies report that pain is still there, but they no longer care about it. It is as though pain has again become an external quality like other sensations, something that can be contemplated dispassionately rather than as a condition of the self. Here, perhaps, is the mind-body puzzle in one of its purest forms.

Opium, opiates, opioids

Modern medicine has at its disposal an arsenal of drugs which are important modifiers of pain; prominent among which are chemicals known as *opiates*. At least fifty-five centuries ago, around 3500 B.C., the Sumerians used the Eurasian poppy (*Papaver somniferum*) to reduce the discomforts of dysentery, an application still practiced in modern medicine. It is not clear when its effectiveness as a pain-killer, or *analgesic*, was first discovered, but it is known that medicinal use of the poppy was made in ancient Egypt, Persia, and Greece. Later it was brought to India and eventually to China. Apparently its misuse there as an addictive drug did not begin until the seventeenth century when the Western habit of smoking reached the Far East. Instead of smoking tobacco, the Chinese began to smoke opium.

By the nineteenth century, Europe exported enormous quantities of opium to China. When the Chinese government threatened to block further imports of the drug, the Opium Wars of 1839–1858 forced China to continue the trade.

Opium is obtained by drying the juice extracted from the unripe seed pods of the poppy. Its effect is to induce a state of relaxation, drowsiness, and euphoria. It contains a number of active ingredients called *alkaloids*, among them *morphine, codeine, papaverine*, and others. When morphine was isolated, it was found to be a powerful analgesic. It has been the treatment of choice for pain from battle injuries in every war since the American Civil War. Soon other alkaloids with similar properties were discovered. These *opiates* all turned out to have very similar chemical structures. The most powerful among them, *etorphine,* is between five thousand and ten thousand times more potent than morphine.

Among the opiates is a group of substances called *antagonists.* Their structure is again very similar to that of morphine, but their effect is drastically different. In very small doses these substances are able to counteract the analgesic effect of morphine and similar opiates. One such chemical is *naloxone.* By itself it is slightly toxic, but its effects are rather minor. When given with morphine, the latter is rendered virtually ineffective as a pain-killer.

Here, then, is the first part of the opium puzzle: The opiates are highly specific analgesics, some being effective in minute doses. However, other opiates, the antagonists like naloxone, cancel almost completely the analgesic effects of morphine. All opiates, the analgesics as well as their antagonists, have strikingly similar molecular shapes.

These facts suggest that naloxone, rather than altering or otherwise neutralizing morphine, may *pose* as morphine without having the analgesic properties of morphine. The fact that morphine molecules are then unable to act suggests further that there may be a limited number of locations in the brain which are able to *receive* these molecules, and if these *sites* are blocked by the ineffectual naloxone, then morphine molecules find themselves with no places to go.

All evidence seemed to point to the existence of such highly specific *receptor sites* in the central nervous system. They were called *opiate receptors.* The supposition was that protein molecules distributed over the neural membrane may have just the right shape for one of the opiate molecules to become attached, but that they are unable to distinguish morphine from its antagonists. If morphine becomes attached, it will act as a neurotransmitter (see pages 52–53), and analgesic action will result. The selectivity of such receptor sites would explain how minute quantities of opiates reaching the central nervous system could exert such a powerful and highly specific action, and how a substance like naloxone, by mimicking these opiates, is able to block this action.

The theory of opiate receptors was confirmed in the early seventies by the use of opiates carrying a radioactive element, or *label,* which made it possible to trace their locations in the brain. Opiate receptors were found to be concentrated along the pathways known to be involved in pain conduction—in the spinal cord, the thalamus, and the cerebral cortex.

The confirmation of the opiate receptor theory solved one puzzle but introduced another, even more confounding one: How did a mechanism as delicate and as specific as that of the opium receptors evolve? Was it just an accident, or did evolution anticipate man's discovery of the opium poppy? Both alternatives seemed rather unpalatable.

Another theory now was proposed to solve this new puzzle. Could it be that the central nervous system manufactured its own pain-killers with properties similar to those of the opiates, and that the system of receptors was really designed for *them*? The search was on for these opiate-like brain secretions, the *opioids*.

The story proceeds like a good detective yarn. We mentioned in the last section that electrical stimulation in parts of the brain can reduce pain sensation. In 1976 it was found that when naloxone was administered at the same time, this analgesic action disappeared.[19] The conclusion seemed inescapable: Electrical stimulation caused the release of some opiate-like substances, which can be blocked by naloxone. Another bit of circumstantial evidence was added when it was found that extracts from mouse brain produced in mice effects similar to those caused by opiates, and that furthermore these effects were again reduced by the administration of naloxone.

Meanwhile the first brain *opioids* were isolated and identified in 1975. John Hughes and his collaborators at the University of Aberdeen in Scotland found two substances they called *enkephalins*,[20] small chain molecules, each consisting of five amino acids. (Amino acids are the building blocks from which the large protein molecules are constructed.) Soon other opioids were found and were called *endorphins*. They consist of somewhat longer amino-acid sequences, but are still much smaller than proteins. When minute doses of enkephalins or endorphins were injected directly into the brains of experimental animals, they showed morphine-like analgesic properties. It has been proposed that the mechanism by which morphine as well as the brain opioids achieve their effect involves the suppression of *substance P*, mentioned in the last section as a possible pain-specific transmitter substance.

The newly found enkephalins, endorphins, and substance P belong to a growing class of chemicals called *neuropeptides*. These substances (with names like *neurotensin, somatostatin, bombesin*, and others) carry out a bewildering variety of functions, including control of hormone release by the pituitary gland, control of emotional states, and transmitter functions in the nervous system. If the preceding sentence sounds vague and complicated, it only conveys the status of a new, exciting, but still very confused field. Peptides, often the same ones, are found in the hypothalamus, the pituitary gland, the cerebral cortex, and even in the intestines. This has given rise to a new way of looking at hormonal function and has led endocrinologists to speak of the *"brain-gut axis."*

Some of the brain peptides are believed to act as *hormones* by being circulated in the bloodstream, some as neurotransmitters, merely crossing the narrow gap between communicating neurons. The two modes have been compared to a radio broadcast and a telephone conversation, respectively. In the hormonal role, as in radio communication, the message is *broadcast*—that is, disseminated widely—but requires very special equipment (*receivers* and *receptors*) to be picked up. Synaptic transmission, by contrast, like a telephone conversation is between two stations over a private line.

The hormonal, or endocrine, role of the brain is an aspect that must be considered in addition to the classical picture of the *neural network,* in which action potentials are carried over an incredibly delicate and complex circuitry of fibers. Throughout the same system there may be many simultaneous broadcasts of chemical messages to widely distributed and finely tuned receptors.

In Chapter 2 I discussed some of the early ideas on brain function. I pointed out (see page 38) how anatomists as far back as Galen in the second century A.D. attributed brain action to its fluid rather than its solid portions, and how the fluid-filled ventricles remained the center of attention among anatomists until about the end of the Renaissance.

Not unlike the city of Venice, which is bathed on all sides by the sea, the brain is surrounded and cushioned by the cerebrospinal fluid and invaded by a system of canals connecting the larger pools, the *ventricles.* Apart from serving as a shock absorber and perhaps as an internal "sewer" that carries waste products away from the brain, little importance has been attributed to this system in modern times. However, something like the old *pneuma theory* may yet be revived. We know that the abovementioned *peptides* occur in high concentrations in the cerebrospinal fluid, and that peptides administered artificially into the ventricles produce immediate behavioral consequences. Some physiologists believe that the cerebrospinal fluid provides the neuropeptides with transport and rapid access to widely separated portions in the brain, particularly the so-called *limbic system* which surrounds the ventricles and is generally held responsible for the control of emotions.

5

MIND: THE OTHER SIDE OF THE COIN

. . . But the mind in apprehending also experiences sensations which, properly speaking, are qualities of the mind alone. These sensations are projected by the mind so as to clothe appropriate bodies in external nature. Thus the bodies are perceived as with qualities which in reality do not belong to them, qualities which in fact are purely the offspring of the mind. Thus nature gets credit which should in truth be reserved for ourselves: the rose for its scent; the nightingale for its song; and the sun for its radiance. The poets are entirely mistaken. They should address their lyrics to themselves, and should turn them into odes of self-congratulation on the excellency of the human mind. Nature is a dull affair, soundless, scentless, colourless; merely the hurrying of material, endlessly, meaninglessly.

—A. N. WHITEHEAD, Science and the Modern World

. . . a mind that could know the object-world without any error would know nothing at all.

—ALAIN (ÉMILE AUGUSTE CHARTIER), The Gods

The lengthy midsection of this book has been devoted mostly to facts about the physical brain. Without losing sight of these, we will now turn to some of the phenomena we generally associate with *mind*. The borderline is not sharp. We mentioned consciousness and sensations in Chapter 4, especially in connection with our discussions of pain and of the reticular activating system (RAS). In this chapter we will continue to refer back to various parts of the brain, but the emphasis will be on the mind.

I hope what follows will dispel the notion that questions of mind are solely the province of philosophy. Whatever philosophers have to say about mind, they must become aware of new findings in the neurosciences as well as of principles of physics that have a direct bearing on the subject. To ignore these is to run the risk of producing irrelevant philosophies.

I must make it clear that my aim will be not to come up with new answers to the mind-body dilemma but to take the liberty of criticizing some old ones and point in the direction that new empirical facts seem to suggest. A new vision, consistent with our deepening understanding of the human nervous system and the physical universe at large, will emerge slowly, probably after many more false starts.

We will begin by looking at those processes which go beyond our concept of the sensory-motor brain. These include, on the one hand, sensory inputs which are elaborated to varying degrees by the manipulative mind without necessarily leading to motor action, and, on the other hand, motor actions that emerge spontaneously or as a result of cerebral activities generally described as *thought*.

Perception: the thinking man's filter

It is one thing to look passively, disinterestedly at a pattern of moving clouds. It is quite another thing to view them with a weatherman's eye, examining them for signs presaging this or that weather pattern, or just to imagine them to be gargoyles or rabbits. The first case of *seeing* we may be tempted to interpret in a simpleminded fashion: Light reflected by the clouds enters the eye, is focused on the retina, where a neural pattern is created and transmitted to the visual cortex. There the neural code simply reports "white, irregular shapes slowly drifting across a blue background." The second set of circumstances is more often referred to as *perception*. What is the difference? It has been stated that the first is the province of the physiologist, the second of the psychologist. In one case we can follow and analyze the physical processes that go on in the brain, in the other we can't. Or so it was thought. As it turns out, we may have been overly optimistic in the first case and too pessimistic in the second.

When we examined the visual system in Chapter 4, we found that the processes of information flow from receptors to the brain are much more complex than we had anticipated. What we thought was a simple relay station—the lateral geniculate nucleus (LGN)—becomes a place where the messages from the eyes are mixed with the echoes from the cortex. In this way the cortex reaches out to the periphery, intercepting the incoming messages, filtering and altering its own input. Thus fact and fancy are interwoven on this "internal retina," and the two cases cited in the preceding paragraph are perhaps only different mixes of the same basic ingredients.

Let us examine now some specific examples in which seeing is evidently more than just translating light patterns into neural patterns. It is a well-known fact that localized regions of visual defects can go unnoticed. The perceived visual patterns surrounding blind spots (scotomas) are extended through the nonseeing area by the perceiving brain. In 1975 P. Tynan and R. Sekuler[1] of Northwestern University in Evanston, Illinois, showed that such visual *phantoms*, as they are called, can also appear in portions of the visual field that are served by a healthy, functioning retina and visual cortex. In this experiment a pattern of alternating dark and bright vertical stripes was displayed on an oscilloscope screen. The pattern was masked across the middle by a horizontal strip of black tape. When the pattern was moved horizontally, subjects would get the impression that the bright bands continued across the obscured center.

Similar effects of *pattern completion* are known in hearing. When an *obvious* short word is deleted in a recorded sentence and replaced by noise, subjects report hearing the original sentence. Thus "Go (noise) the store" is heard as "Go to the store."

These are clearly cases in which the mind interprets reality and, in doing so, modifies it. A somewhat different type of modification occurs in the case of the Necker cube, shown in Fig. 5.1. As we look at this picture, we have a distinct impression of a three-dimensional figure. We *know* which side of the cube is toward us, which away from us. But this situation periodically and quite abruptly changes, with the cube assuming different positions in space. We ask, what is changing in the perception of this simple figure? The pattern of black lines on the white surface in front of us is always the same. It is flat, favoring neither one interpretation nor the other. But something additional is supplied by the observer. He is made more acutely aware of that addi-

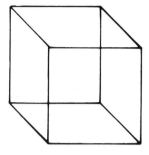

5.1 *Necker cube*

tional element in his perception because of the competing interpretations that keep alternating.

We encounter a similar situation in contemplating Fig. 5.2. Here the different interpretations stem from the ambiguity between what is the figure and what the background. Accordingly, you will see either a vase or two human heads facing each other. As in the case of the Necker cube, the two interpretations are mutually exclusive, and the perception switches spontaneously from one to the other.

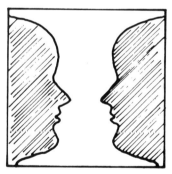

5.2 *The figure-ground dilemma*

The next two examples are somewhat different. When shown either Figs. 5.3 or 5.4, a subject generally doesn't know what to make of them; they are just black lines on a white background. But his perception will change drastically when he is told that Fig. 5.3 shows a military guard and a guard dog seen through an open barracks gate, which they have just passed, and Fig. 5.4 depicts a pair of railroad tracks with a train receding into the distance.

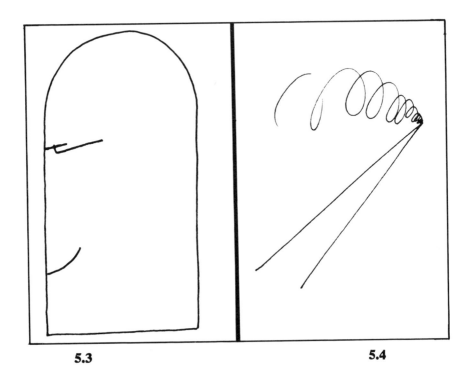

5.3   **5.4**

Again we ask, what has changed in our perception? The same lines are projected on the retina, and the neural messages produced there presumably are the same as before. They will continue to serve as a check on the reality before us, but this is probably where the similarity with the previous response ends. The existence of the elaborate pathways "coming down" from the cortex makes it seem likely that the pattern appearing on the "inner retina" of the LGN is already very different. (We are reminded here of the discussion of the visual pathway and the thalamic relay nuclei in Chapter 4.) There may even be hints of the figure of a guard outside the barracks wall, or the continuation of the dog (Fig. 5.5). Somewhere else there is perhaps a suggestion of the sound of the guard's footfall. Our mind is free to supply these sensations as long as they are not too much in conflict with the reality of which we are constantly being reminded.

Look again at the picture of the railroad tracks. Where the smoke starts, we can almost make out a suggestion of the train. We have the feeling that we could see details of the engine or the caboose if only we could magnify the picture. In Fig. 5.6 we have done just that. Here is an enlarged picture of that portion of Fig. 5.4 where the "tracks"

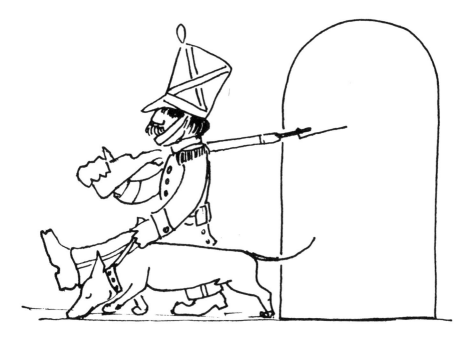

5.5 *What you didn't see before*

meet the horizon and the locomotive belches black smoke. But now the illusion is gone. We see only an irregular black shape that has no resemblance to a train.

I believe the vanishing of the illusion has to do with the fact that what we see is now too grossly incompatible with the previous interpretation. In this case reality gets the upper hand. We can think of the fantasizing brain as attempting to wrest control over our perceptions away from the sensory input, while the senses keep the flow of imagination in check and anchor our perceptions in reality. If the anchor chain breaks, we are adrift with our dreams and hallucinations. If the sensory control is too powerful, our perceptions are dull, unimaginative. Twenty-four centuries ago Democritus described this seesaw battle in his famous dialogue between the mind and the senses. First, the mind chides the senses, pointing out that their qualities of color or taste are only matters of convention. The senses answer:

Ah, wretched intellect, you get your evidence only as we give it to you, and yet you try to overthrow us. That overthrow will be your downfall.

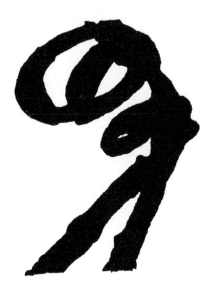

5.6 *Where is the train now?*

Another example shows this conflict between fact and fancy. Figure 5.7 will be seen by most observers as a mosaic of squares of different shades of gray. Now look at Fig. 5.8 on the next page. The same picture is reproduced but this time slightly out of focus. Most of us will recognize the face almost immediately. The interpretive brain has no difficulty manipulating the pattern to form the familiar face. But why are we unable to do the same with the picture on page 161, even after being told what it represents? The answer lies in the fact that the strong sensory reality of the sharply delineated squares in Fig. 5.7 distracts the perceiving mind and prevents it from imposing its fancy on the pattern received. With Fig. 5.8, because of the blurred outlines, the mind is free to bend sensory reality to conform to its fantasy, in this case the one most compatible with reality.

The picture of perception presented here emphasizes the role played by imagery and, more generally, by information being reflected from higher centers. Not all psychologists, however, acknowledge that old information stored in the brain is a major ingredient in perception. James J. Gibson of Cornell University in Ithaca, New York, believed that perception is a *direct* process, involving a minimum of cerebral transactions. Similarly, in *gestalt* psychology it is held that the properties and significance of every perceived object are contained in the direct stimulus that object engenders. "A fruit says 'Eat me'; water says

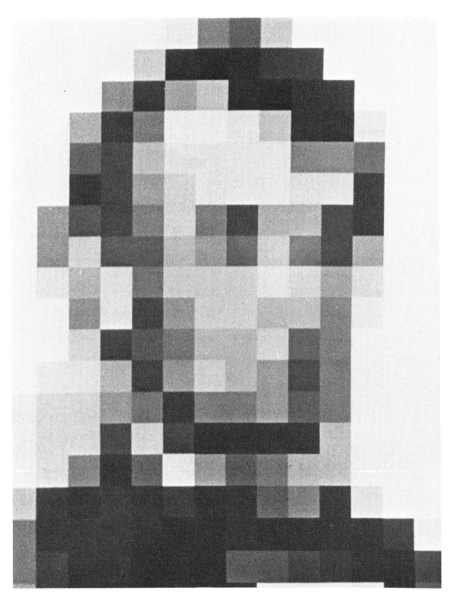

5.7 *What is it (in focus)? (This photograph was produced and kindly supplied by Leon D. Harmon at Bell Laboratories.)*

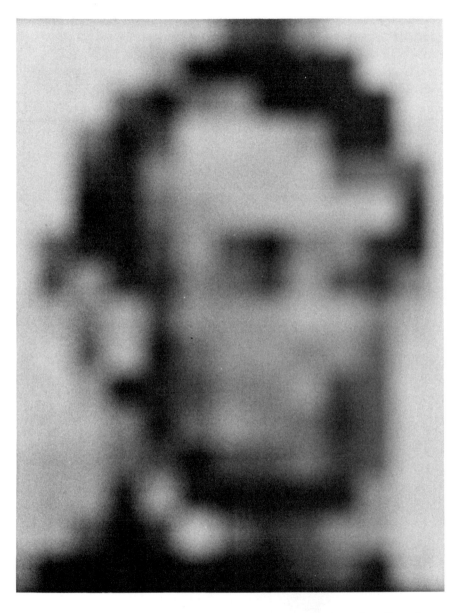

5.8 *Out of focus. (A blurred print made from the preceding figure)*

'Drink me'; thunder says 'Fear me'; and woman says 'Love me' " is the way Kurt Koffka[3] describes perceptual immediacy. Gibson, in his *theory of affordances,* assigns a minor role to memory and learning, pointing out that the "affordances" of an object are intrinsic in the stimulus. Here are some examples Gibson gives of affordances that are evident through *direct* perception:

> A rigid object with a sharp dihedral angle, an edge, affords cutting and scraping. It is a *knife* . . .

> An elongated elastic object like a fiber, thread, thong, or rope affords knotting, binding, lashing, and weaving . . .

> A graspable rigid object of moderate size and weight affords throwing. It may be a missile or only an object for play, a *ball* . . .[4]

The controversy over whether perception is direct (à la Gibson) or indirect has some of the earmarks of a psychological *hang-up,* not unlike those in neuroscience discussed in Chapter 3. In all likelihood both viewpoints contain some truth, at least some of the time. Our perception (and fear) of heights appears from experiments with human infants to be direct.[5] It does not depend on previous experiences of falling, or on warnings, or on other unpleasant associations. We must conclude that it is of genetic origin. Our perception of a red traffic light as a signal to stop the car is clearly a *learned* response, and yet it appears to be as immediate as the sudden appearance of a chasm in front of us or the thunder's "Fear me."

But perception does not always stop there, especially when the perceived object evokes conflict or puzzlement or emotion. The ensuing interplay between senses and *mind* is perception of a different kind and can no longer be characterized as *direct.* The content of what is sensed directly may be manipulated, distorted, in part emphasized, in part suppressed, and new features may be substituted. If I understand Alain correctly, these are the "errors" to which he refers in the quotation on page 154, and which we have seen at work in some of the pictorial examples given above. Without manipulation of some of these raw sense data we would indeed "know nothing at all."

Perception rarely involves just *one* of our senses. You feel a breeze on your face due to various skin sensors there. At the same time, you hear it and you see its effect as movement on the water or in the trees. The sensation of moving air is a harmonious confluence of many senses. If any one of these were absent or grossly mismatched, our perception would seem *unreal*. There is a doctrine in psychology called the *theory of cognitive dissonance*,[6] according to which the mind will make every attempt to achieve *consonance* by finding *explanations* for sensory or cognitive discrepancies. But sometimes the discrepancies are too severe. Imagine hearing a howling storm, but feeling and seeing only a gentle breeze. Sensory mismatches like this are startling and are common devices used by makers of horror movies. But the events of everyday life are perceived as particular combinations of different sensations. Such characteristic composites are sometimes called *sensory schemata*. Introspection leads me to believe that events are stored in memory as schemata, and that thinking of an event "brings to mind" the same harmonious combination of sensations. We will see how the concept of a sensory schema is particularly useful in trying to understand the initiation and control of motor action.

Our discussion of perception would not be complete without a look at the efferent side of the brain. Motor pathways are inextricably involved in sensory perception. We have seen that sensors are built into every part of our action apparatus—the muscles, the tendons, the joints—and that, conversely, the somatosensory cortex, the locus of our body sensations, borders on and probably talks across to the motor cortex. Thus actions produce sensations, and sensations cause actions. Simulated action—that is, the *thought* of action—makes us think also of the sensations such actions would engender. A "train of thought" generally contains both of these ingredients in a continuous feedback, one reinforcing the other. This might be a runaway situation were it not for the fact that new and different sense impressions continue to stream in, each seeking the attention of the central nervous system. Thus we are continuously *distracted*. But in the natural sensory isolation of sleep, or the artificial sensory deprivation produced in isolation experiments, these feedback loops can lead to dreams in one case and full-blown hallucinatory experiences in another.

We set out to talk about mind, and we are back discussing the body. This may simply be the predilection of a physicist in these matters. We must not leave the subject of perception without saying a word about that very controversial and much-talked-about topic: extrasensory perception, or ESP.

What we have been discussing above is literally *extra-sensory*, since the sensory messages are only a fraction, the bare beginning of perception. The other part is supplied by the brain itself. Not only does it elaborate on the hard facts which the senses report, it also computes ahead and anticipates much of what is about to happen. It does this on the basis of what it has just learned, and on the basis of a lifetime's accumulation of facts and associations. We would normally not call this *extrasensory* or *clairvoyance*, but, strictly speaking, that is exactly what it is. I look at a scene and I can predict some future events. If I see a car speeding out of control, I can foresee the crash. An event can also be surmised from cues that are only indirectly connected with the event. I know that a door has opened somewhere from the perception of a draft of air or a change in the acoustics of the room. Nobody will dispute these effects. Let it be understood, then, that the claim of ESP is something quite different. It is the purported flow of *new* information from the world that is exterior to the subject by means other than his senses. At this point, traditional scientists and parapsychologists generally part company.

Action

Recall for a moment our discussion in Chapter 4 in which we distinguished between actions that were clearly precipitated by immediate sensory events (ducking when an object is thrown at you) and an act of *caprice,* that is, a sudden act whose immediate cause does not lie in events external to the individual. We had postponed discussion of this second category of events because it involves protracted and poorly understood neural processes that are generally labelled *mental.*

There now exist interesting new neurological data on such spontaneous voluntary actions. Nothing as dramatic as a man jumping off a bridge, but merely the sudden, voluntary flexing of a finger by a subject told to do so "at will."

I am referring to a series of experiments by H. H. Kornhuber and collaborations in Germany in 1976. They recorded electrical signals from various points on the scalps of human volunteers. These *electroencephalograms* (EEG's) were taken while the subjects performed various motor tasks. In one experiment[7] subjects were instructed to flex the index finger of the right hand suddenly, but at times of their own choosing. An electrical signal was also obtained from the muscle controlling the finger, thereby giving the experimenters precise markers of the times when the movement was initiated.

The EEG traces are irregular lines that reflect many things going on

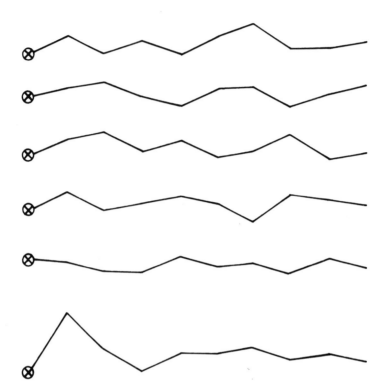

5.9 *Five random traces with a "buried" signal. The last trace is the sum of the five and shows the "unearthed" signal.*

simultaneously in the brain. They are the muffled voices of the active brain, heard faintly through a quarter inch of skullbone. Buried in these traces are the signals that may be related to the decision-making process that leads up to the finger flexing and the eventual commands issued by the cortex. By adding many such traces and averaging them, we can cull repeatable and hence meaningful features out of the noise. To do this it is necessary to align the traces properly, that is, to have a time marker in each, and thereby define corresponding instances in each of the traces. The principle is illustrated in the following diagram (Fig. 5.9). Here five mostly random traces are shown with their markers (X) aligned. The last trace shows what happens when we add the five traces. Note that the original traces look quite irregular, but their sum shows a distinct peak following the time marker. Something clearly happens right after the (X), but in the individual traces that "signal" is buried in the noise.

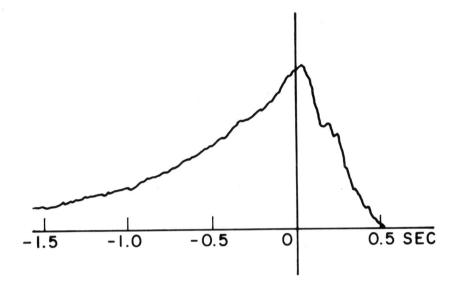

5.10 *Readiness potential. The rise starts over a second before the voluntary act. (After Kornhuber)*

In the experiments described above, the time marker was the first electrical signal picked up from the flexor muscle. The decision to flex must evidently have occurred before the marker. Kornhuber and his team therefore used what they called *time reversed averaging*, that is, they averaged the EEG traces just before the time markers. The results for an electrode attached to the top of the scalp are shown in Fig. 5.10. In this trace we see a gradual rise in voltage, beginning as much as 1.5 seconds before the time marker which is time zero. The rise is interpreted as an increase in cortical activity.

Similar traces were observed with electrodes in different scalp locations. Two features of these curves are of particular interest to us here. Remember (see page 140) that commands for voluntary action start in the Betz cells of the motor cortex and descend through the pyramidal tract into the spinal cord, where they trigger motoneurons. The earliest signals announcing the voluntary flexing of the right forefinger should therefore come from someplace in the left motor cortex (the left motor cortex controls the right side of the body), that is, a region in front of the central sulcus (Fig. 4.21). And since the pathways conducting these signals downward are fast, we could expect the EEG traces from there to show the incipient action perhaps a tenth of a second before it actually takes place, but not much earlier. Instead, Kornhuber's data show that something begins to happen a full second or more before the action. The other interesting finding is that these early signals of impending action are picked up not just from the motor cortex. A considerable part of this early activity occurs behind the central sulcus, in the *somatosensory cortex!*

The neural dynamics of such spontaneous voluntary action is evidently quite different from actions triggered by external stimuli. We can't afford to take a full second to react to some emergencies. We have learned that many stimulus-reaction pairs are "wired-in" as reflexes at the level of the spinal cord, requiring no time-consuming decision-making from above. But even when the cortex is involved, the times between stimulus and action can be quite short. If a subject is instructed to push a button as soon as he sees a light flashing on or hears a buzzer, reaction times are of the order of one tenth of a second. This is about ten times faster than the slow buildup of activity observed in Kornhuber's data.

What, then, goes on in the brain during that relatively long stretch of one second preceding this spontaneous voluntary action? We cannot be sure, but we will make a guess. The flexing of the forefinger, like any action, is accompanied by a variety of sensory responses, visual and skin responses, plus the internal senses of muscle, joint, and tendon. Together they constitute a sensory pattern, a *schema*. But, unlike the one discussed in the preceding section—seeing and hearing the wind and feeling it on your face—this one involves one's own actions. Let us call it a *proprioceptive schema.*

It is this sensory event that I think must be invoked prior to spontaneous voluntary actions. *Thinking* about the action means thinking of the various sensory reports that normally result from the action—the proprioceptive schema. I suspect that the early activity coming from sensory cortex in Kornhuber's data reflects this phenomenon. The gradual buildup we see in Fig. 5.10 would then result from a feedback, perhaps from the adjacent motor cortex which is tuned to that same action. The spillover of the growing somatosensory activity across the central sulcus into the motor region will eventually precipitate the action itself.

I want to emphasize that the details of what I have described here are speculative. The following, however, are known facts: The somatosensory cortex and the motor cortex join at the central sulcus and communicate across the boundary. Spontaneous voluntary actions are preceded by cortical activity in the somatosensory cortex as well as the motor cortex. In the Kornhuber experiment, this activity takes about a second to build up to its peak value, at which time the intended action occurs.

We have raised before the question of how we control ongoing motor action by using sensory information to correct for errors in judgment, and generally making the performance conform to some precept of the action. This does not apply, of course, to actions that are carried out so rapidly there is no time for feedback control.

But let us consider a protracted action such as lifting a cup of tea to one's lips, being careful to direct the motion to the right target and not spilling any liquid on the way. Or, better yet, think of bowing a string instrument, which involves extremely delicate muscular control, guided by the *feel* of the bow as well as the resulting sound. I want to propose an alternative to the theory of control by *efference copy* which, as we have seen (pages 143, 144), had two shortcomings. The supposition was that a copy of the set of motor commands is kept somewhere in the brain, and performance is compared with this *efference copy*. As I mentioned, we know of no location where such a copy might be kept, and we do not understand how the sensory feedback resulting from the action could be matched against the original motor commands. They are in *different languages*.

If voluntary action begins as a proprioceptive schema, as we had supposed in connection with Kornhuber's experiments, then the blueprint for the action and the sensory reports would not only occur in the same location, the somatosensory cortex, but they would be in the same language, hence directly comparable.

Sketchpad in the head

An artist, before starting a new painting, usually begins with a sketch. The dynamics of this process is intriguing. An idea originates in the brain of the artist and is *projected,* made concrete on a piece of paper, only to be examined and judged by the same brain that was its source. Changes are made, features are added, and again the concrete results are scrutinized by the creating mind. Eventually the artist may be satisfied to advance from sketch to canvas, or he may tear up the sketch in dismay and decide it's time to go fishing. But without the sketch the artist's ability to judge his own ideas would be limited. Similarly, a poet would be lost without pencil and paper, and a composer without a keyboard.

Language often serves a similar function. Talking to oneself is not a mental aberration but often serves to clarify one's thoughts. Piaget observed that the use of language in children begins not as a form of communication intended for others, but as a soliloquy. Children think aloud, telling themselves what they already know.

The artist, the poet, the musician would have a difficult time without the means of external storage and contemplation of their ideas. But they would not be entirely lost. We have the ability to conjure up, and for a limited time to hold and examine, visual, auditory, and tactile images. This is the faculty of mental *simulation,* which we have already discussed. We can also call to mind the sensory schemata that go with particular actions. The musician and the athlete know that *thinking* about an exercise is the next best thing to doing it.

The mechanisms for such processes are the most challenging and the most obscure. How and where are images created? If we take a hint from the above examples, we might guess that thinking involves schemata that are conceived in the brain, most likely in the neocortex, projected to a more peripheral level—an *internal sketchpad,* so to speak—and then reexamined at the higher level. Such a continuous feedback loop is a plausible model for thought, but we must emphasize that we are now making guesses. Let us see how such a model might fit in with what we have learned about the brain so far.

In Chapter 2 the section entitled "Neurons: the way in and the way out" contains a sketch of the basic architecture of a brain (Fig. 2.8 on page 47). This sketch shows afferent pathways ascending via sensory relay stations to the cerebral cortex, and efferent pathways which descend via motor relays to the muscles. Reflex arcs bypass this larger arc by linking receptors directly with effectors, mostly through the spinal cord.

Note that this system has no internal loops. Whatever enters through the sensory channels, if it causes any effect at all, will exit on the motor side.

In Fig. 5.11 I have reproduced the same diagram with some modifications. The top of the hierarchy of neurons is now split into a sensory part (B_1) and a motor part (B_2). In B_1 are the sensory areas of the cortex, including the somatosensory cortex, where most sensory information concerning the body is collected. In B_2 is the motor cortex,

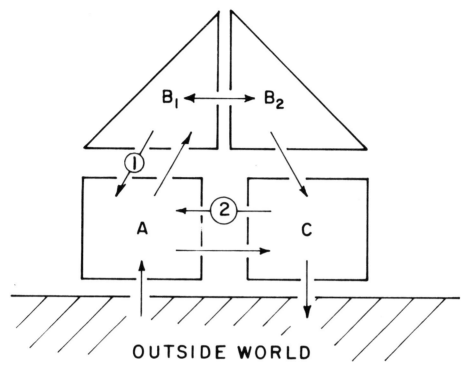

5.11 *The nervous system. A simple overview with some complications.*

where commands are issued to the skeletal muscles. The central sulcus is the dividing line between the two, and the double arrow represents the presumed two-way communication across the boundary. The squares, A and C, stand for subcortical areas, separated again according to their location on the afferent (A) or efferent side (C) of the nervous system. Square A thus contains the sensory relays in the thalamus, but also the ascending sensory pathways in the spinal cord. Square C contains the efferent motor pathways, including the pyramidal tract and the system of motoneurons in the spinal cord. The principal new features in this diagram are the arrows labeled 1 and 2. Arrow 1 denotes the *corticofugal* pathways, by which parts of the sensory cortex react back on sensory relays in the thalamus, thus creating a loop of activity between A and B$_1$, Arrow 2 represents the proprioceptive feedback: sensory information about body movements and positions including the reports from the muscle spindles described in Chapter 4. A further complication comes from the fact that the brain can modify its owns somatosensory input by way of the system of gamma motoneurons and intrafusal muscles. This is another example of centrifugal or corticofugal control.

The block diagram of the nervous system in Fig. 5.11 is still highly oversimplified. Many brain centers, such as the reticular activating system (RAS), are simply overlooked here or lumped together with other parts. Still, the model that is implied by this figure is vastly more complex in its function than its more primitive counterpart on page 171. The added complexity, moreover, is achieved with relatively little added structure. What makes the enormous difference is the addition of the feedback loops. The fact that raw sense data are now mixed with analyzed data to become new sense data raises the complexity of the neural dynamics to a degree that cannot be overstated. It introduces a problem which logicians recognize as the problem of *self-reference*, to which we will come back later. It can be compared with standing between two mirrors and seeing an apparently infinite regression of images. Psychologists often tend to shy away from this unwelcome complication and seek ways of avoiding the infinite regression (I know that I know that I know . . .) implied by these structures. The regression, of course, is not *infinite* but only *indefinite*, since the time of perception is finite.

The return paths from the cortex to the thalamic relays (arrow 1 in Fig. 5.11) raises another set of interesting puzzles. As we have seen, every sense except smell has its relay station in the thalamus and its own specific return path from the cortex. What is the nature of these returning messages?

Recall that the part of the thalamus that is concerned with vision, the lateral geniculate nucleus (LGN), preserves some of the character of the retina: Activity is distributed over sheets of neurons which mirror the pattern of light falling on the retina. It is possible that corticofugal messages weave similar patterns on this *inner retina*, as Wolf Singer has called it.[8] This is suggested by the fact that the fibers coming back from the cortex are about as numerous as those going in the opposite directions, and have the same spatial distribution over the sheet of neurons in the relay nucleus. Also there is evidence that the returning messages are *feature specific*; that is, they can enhance, select, and perhaps mimic sensory patterns. Another bit of circumstantial evidence is the finding that in cats, activity in the LGN is heightened during REM sleep, that phase of sleep in which we are supposed to dream. Moreover, this activity was found to be similar in character to that evoked by real visual input.

I would like to suggest an extension of Singer's concept of an "internal retina" to what I called an *"internal sketchpad."* The idea is that sensory patterns are laid down in the LGN by sensory input, but similar patterns may also be sketched there by higher centers. The LGN is a possible location for such a process, but certainly not the only place where this may occur.

If this is a correct picture, then we must explain how the "mind," through processes taking place in the neocortex, is able to evoke stimuli that resemble the features of the imagined object or event. Karl Pribram of the Stanford University School of Medicine speaks of the problem of the *invertible transform* in sensory mapping.[9] The problem can be described by some parallels. Consider a burglar alarm. Here is a system, electronic or otherwise, which flashes a light, sounds a siren, or sends a message to the nearest police station when an act of burglary is committed or about to be committed. The normal flow of events is then: appearance of burglar, detection of burglar, transmission of coded information announcing burglary.

Clearly this transformation is *not* invertible. If I were to cause the alarm at the police station to go off by some other means, this would not smash the windows at a nearby store and cause a man to enter with larcenous intent. Similarly, printing an inflated Dow Jones average on a ticker tape will not turn a sagging stock market around, nor will the sound of music falling on the speaker of a jukebox cause a coin to pop out of the slot. These are all examples of noninvertible transforms.

A little reflection on these and similar examples will convince one that most chains of causally connected events cannot be turned around. There are several reasons for these irreversibilities; some have to do with principles in physics; in general, information is discarded in these transforms and cannot be recovered on the way back.

One example of a process that is readily reversed is the generation of electrical power by cranking a generator. If, instead, the unit is connected to a source of electrical power, it acts as a motor. More interesting from our point of view is the mapping that takes place in the formation of an optical hologram such as the one shown on page 89. The pattern of irregular ripples is obtained by exposing a photographic plate to beams of laser light, one of which was scattered from a small object, in this case the two nude figures. Then by passing similar laser light through the developed photographic plate, the original scene is re-created in full stereo. Again, the process is to some extent invertible: object produces hologram, hologram re-creates object, at least something that looks like it.

Let us go back to something we discussed in Chapter 3: the function of feature detectors in the nervous system. The neural alarm system of an animal that detects danger from the appearance of certain patterns of stimuli is in principle similar to a burglar alarm. And, just as the burglar alarm is irreversible, it is difficult to see how the *thought* of an event could cause the appearance of the event, or something like it, in our sensory channels. And yet this is what we are suggesting in our interpretation of the role of the sensory and proprioceptive feedback loops.

Pribram has suggested that something similar to a holographic process may be used in the brain in mapping sensory information, and may account for the brain's apparent ability to invert the process. This theory has many attractive features. It would explain also the distributed character of stored information that we discussed on pages 85–86. The difficulty is I know of no plausible neural mechanism which could carry out the kind of *computing* that would be necessary to produce and invert a hologram in the brain. As a result, the holographic theory has relatively few adherents today.

In 1976 I proposed an alternative mechanism by which sensory processing may be inverted.[10] It makes use of something called the *Alopex process,* which was discovered two years earlier in my laboratory[11] and has been used successfully in connection with another problem. The principles underlying the process are irrelevant here, but I want to bring out some of the features. Alopex is a statistical process. It works on chances and probabilities.

Consider a hypothetical device which has the property that whenever it *sees* a zebra, it will produce some kind of response. But unlike the burglar alarm which has only two states—full alarm when it is tripped and quiet otherwise—our *zebra detector* has a whole range of responses, from quiet (no zebra) to weak (questionable zebra) to strong (no doubt about the presence of a zebra). In Fig. 5.12 a display device, such as a television screen, is *viewed* by the *zebra detector* on the right. The responses from the detector go to a box which in turn controls the television screen, as indicated by the arrows.

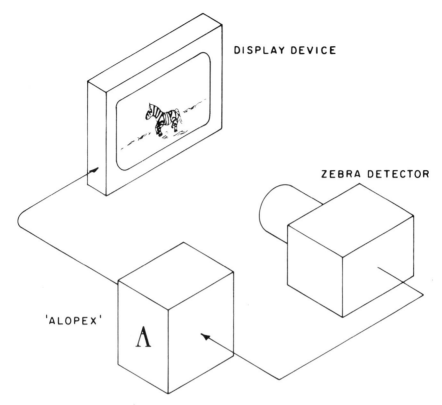

DISPLAY DEVICE

ZEBRA DETECTOR

'ALOPEX'

Λ

5.12 *A feature detector with feedback. Alopex process.*

Let us say that a very fuzzy picture of something resembling a zebra appeared on the screen; hence, a weak response would be given off by the zebra detector. The Alopex device (A) now inverts the process of pattern recognition by causing the picture on the screen to become sharper and more zebra-like. It does this only on the basis of the varying input it receives from the zebra detector: a strong signal when it has done the right thing, a weakened input when it has caused the picture to deteriorate. However, Alopex knows nothing about zebras; if it were connected to a lion detector, it would have made a lion appear on the TV screen. The box (A) is thus a *universal inverter* of the feature-detecting process. How Alopex accomplishes this feat is another story.

The Alopex process is a *primitive* process; it requires only stereotyped repetitions and very little in the way of any complex mechanisms or design. There are many different ways in which it can be accomplished, but the common principle is *feedback control*.

The process has an interesting parallel in the evolution of mimicry in animal forms. Figure 5.13 is a photograph of the *anglerfish*. This

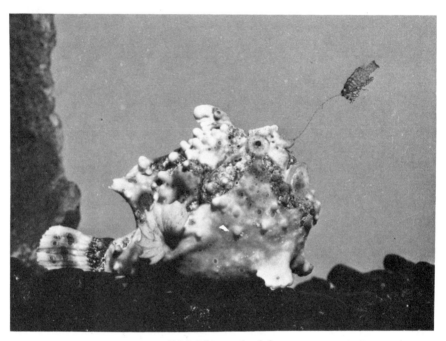

5.13 *The anglerfish*

particular species was described in 1978 by T.W. Pietsch and D.B. Grobecker.[12] The *fish* in the picture looks more like a rock lying on the bottom of the ocean. What looks like a fish is only a structure that evolved at the end of a thin wormlike protuberance coming out of the angler's head. This little "fish" is nothing but a lure that attracts the potential victims of the anglerfish.

What interests us here is how this fishlike protuberance evolved. If we believe in the Darwinian theory of evolution, the slow changes in the animal's DNA that must have brought this about were guided only by the ability of individuals to survive. Many random changes in shape and coloring must have taken place over many millennia. Slowly, very slowly a fin appeared here, an eyespot there, and with every *successful* change it became a better lure and the anglerfish had a better chance to survive.

The parallel between this and the Alopex process may not be too obvious. In both cases the evolving pattern is subject to random events and guided by a feedback process. This, at least, is the model of perception that I wish to propose. The two processes have other fundamental similarities even though one takes place in seconds and the other over millions of years.

Here, then, is another candidate to explain feature-specific feedback in our sensory pathways. In 1976 I showed that a neural Alopex, operating between the cortex and the thalamic relay nuclei, could accomplish substantial feature enhancement in a matter of seconds.[13] The *thought* of a sensory pattern or schema could by this process of inversion insert a faint replica of that pattern into the sensory loop. Once in the loop, it can become progressively reinforced, especially if not contradicted by sensory information. It is possible to account in this way for a whole range of phenomena from sensory enhancement and pattern completion to eidetic imagery, hallucination, and dreaming.

If this interpretation is correct, a dream may begin as a succession of meaningless random patterns of activity on the "internal sketchpad" of the LGN. Some of these patterns may by accident resemble known shapes, just as cloud patterns sometimes assume sudden meaning to us. The cortex will respond to these patterns as if they were sensory inputs. The cortical activity will bear a resemblance to activity evoked there by the real thing. Corticofugal feedback, perhaps through the kind of principles we discussed above, can now act to enhance the peripheral patterns, make them more lifelike. This will produce even stronger central responses. I point again to the analogy with the evolution of the anglerfish, where improved patterns are rewarded with increased chances of survival. In a dream the patterns will not remain stationary since the cortex, through associations, leads from one pattern to the next.

In an earlier chapter we asked where thoughts were made. I favored the notion of strong participation by peripheral systems—sensory or motor systems—as opposed to the idea of an activity that takes place only in the highest centers. We then encountered a similar controversy regarding perception. Here we favored the idea of *central* participation. These two approaches really come down to the proposition that thinking and perceiving are not fundamentally different. They involve the same neural structures and perhaps very similar dynamic principles.

Free will

Few questions about brain functions come so close to touching the core of our self-image as humans as the problem of *volition*, the freedom of *will*.

Freedom is one of our most cherished concepts. Men have died, and others continue to proclaim their willingness to die, in its defense. And yet when we examine the supposed freedom to perform a primitive motor act, such as flexing a finger *at will*, we seem to be at a loss as to the real meaning of the term.

A nineteenth-century materialist would have said that a human is a machine and nothing but a machine, and therefore subject to strict and absolutely deterministic physical laws. The outcome of human actions should be predetermined by the state of the machine and the stimuli impinging on it. Free will must therefore be a delusion. So much for the classical materialist.

Fortunately, we don't have to contend much with this fellow anymore. Few physicists today would subscribe to such a narrow point of view, although in psychology there is still a stubborn residue of the stimulus-response approach championed by B. F. Skinner, and biologists—more than physicists—believe in the ultimate ability of science to *reduce* physical processes to predictable phenomena. We know that nature is full of indeterminacies—we will talk about these later in Chapter 6—though it is not entirely clear how they can ensure our freedom, apart from the fact that it is no longer so easy to rule it out.

In the dualist tradition, freedom of will is achieved by introducing the *mind*. According to Sir John Eccles, the well-known neurophysiologist, who is a believer in the dualist doctrine of mind and body,[14] a conscious, nonphysical entity called *mind*, separate and independent of the brain, is able to exert its influence on the brain, thereby expressing its will. Such control, while it cannot be ruled out, encounters some serious difficulties with known physical laws. It has been called, not inappropriately, a kind of *internal psychokinesis*.

Eccles attempts to make this strange phenomenon more plausible by having the physical system—in this case, circuits of neurons in the brain—so delicately poised that only a minute influence is required to produce the desired effect. Still, the influence is nonphysical, and it is like explaining the birth of an illegitimate child by saying that it was "such a small baby."

I have sketched below a somewhat simplified version of Eccles's scheme. Here are some of the same principal features of the brain that I showed in Fig. 2.15 on page 63: the two halves of the cortex with the two-way connection between them (the *corpus callosum*), the afferent sensory and efferent motor pathways linking each brain half with the opposite half of the body and outside world. All of this, the physical brain and the rest of the physical universe, Eccles calls "World 1." The *conscious self* is a separate entity called "World 2," which communicates directly with the dominant (the left) brain half. Freedom of action is achieved by the "consciously willed influences" of World 2 over World 1. In this way World 1 is relieved of its machine-like progression from state to predestined state.

But how does World 2 make *its* choices? We can presume that it, too, is governed by certain dynamic rules, which involve motivation,

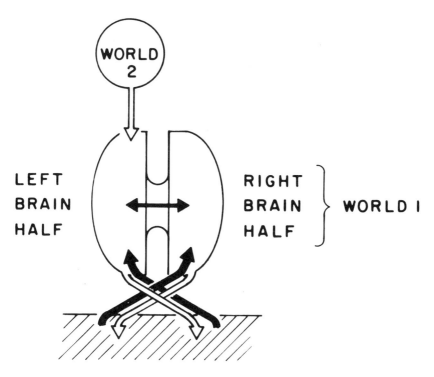

5.14 *Eccles's World 1 and World 2*

drives, emotions, and the like. The dynamics may have a certain looseness, just as the physical laws that govern World 1 have their indeterminacies. But is that freedom? If it were, then Eccles could have ascribed freedom to the brain itself. If it makes no sense to say that the brain has the freedom to impose its will upon itself, then this reasoning must apply equally to World 2. And so we are forced to postulate another world, to liberate World 2 from its mechanisms, and then another and another, each getting its cues from the one above, the last one in that infinite regression being the only one which is really free.

It is perhaps only a step from there to the notion that there is a highest spirit in that hierarchy, the ultimate authority, World Infinity: God.

The traditional concept of freedom thus leads to a paradox. I say that I act freely if my actions are determined by my motivations, my drives, my pleasure. If some external influence interferes with these, then I say that my freedom is restricted. But a dualist would have it that the undisturbed functioning of my brain is *not* free because it is preordained by its own dynamics (which includes drives, needs, etc.). He would impose another will on it (that of World 2). The dualist's dilemma is that his notion of a body's freedom is *freedom from itself*, which leads to the absurd situation pictured above.

We may ask whether contradictory requirements have been included in our traditional concept of freedom. A tentative listing of these is as follows:

(1) the absence of external coercion and control,
(2) the ability to participate in the control of one's surroundings,
(3) the power of determining one's own behavior, and
(4) the sensation of freedom.

Of these requirements (1) and (2) can readily be defined and be reasonably well satisfied. The fourth may be a by-product of the others. I will come back to that point later. The real difficulty lies with the third requirement, because it implies a split between the willing and the acting self. It leads us straight into the dualist trap. It would be nice if we could just dispense with this requirement. If we could, then our freedom would be the same as that of a computer after the RUN button is pushed: It is off and running, free of external control, free to affect the environment with its decisions. Ah, but does it *sense* freedom of action? Unfortunately, nobody can prove that it doesn't. Dropping requirement (3) thus means that we may have to share freedom with

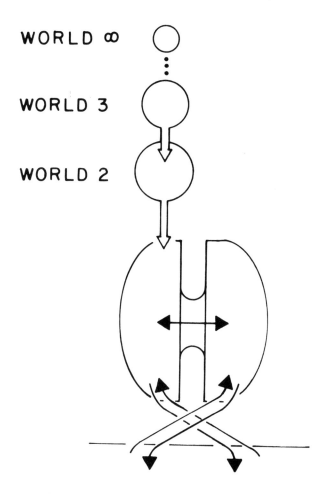

WORLD ∞

WORLD 3

WORLD 2

5.15 *World 1, World 2, . . . World Infinity*

many inanimate natural systems (a spontaneously decaying atom of radium has that freedom) as well as with our more sophisticated machines. Whether this type of freedom still holds interest for us is a matter of taste.

Let us refer back to the experiment we described on page 165, the *voluntary* flexing of a finger. To recapitulate briefly: Subjects were asked to flex the index finger of the right hand suddenly and at times of their own choosing. Electrodes recorded brain activity at various locations and the exact instant of muscle action. The startling finding[15] was that activity in the brain began to rise noticeably as much as a full second before the supposedly deliberate, voluntary action.

We now face this dilemma: If we place the act of "willing" at the beginning of the rising EEG trace (Fig. 5.10, page 167), then introspection tells us that we have been unaware of this slowly growing "decision" for sudden action. But a will without awareness appears to be paradoxical.

What then is the nature of that early rising signal? If it is not the process of willing itself, then perhaps it is preparatory to it. It has been called *readiness potential*. But if it reflects some preparation, then something must know ahead of time what I am about to decide. This would seem to make the subsequent act a foregone conclusion rather than a voluntary act, or else it violates the principle of causality which says that an event (my willing) cannot be the cause of another event which precedes it (the readiness potential). We may well be led to conclude that free will is indeed a delusion, that "autonomous man," to use B. F. Skinner's expression, is a myth.

But what about my *sensation* of free will, that distinct knowledge that I am exercising a discretionary power? In the English language the word *pleasure* can be used as a synonym for free will. It is perhaps the pleasure derived from the resolution of a conflict that gives me the feeling of having made a choice freely.

But sensations have a way of eluding attempts to localize them precisely in time. We talked on pages 98–99 about experiments by Benjamin Libet which showed that the "conscious" sensation of a touch stimulus is delayed by something like half a second. The same thing is true for the sensation of pain: If your hand touches a hot stove, it is withdrawn by a fast reflex long before the slow signal of burning pain is received in the brain. But afterwards you will have the feeling that the act of withdrawing the hand was in response to the pain. The pain sensation and the sensation of voluntariness in withdrawing the hand are both *referred* in time to the overt action itself, of which the nervous system is informed through various channels: you see the hand jerking back and you feel the motion through sensors in your joints and skin. Similarly, the sensation of free will in *voluntarily* flexing your index finger is referred to the instant you feel and see it move. In truth, the sensation may not have occurred until after the act. It is possible that the *conscious* part of the act of willing is the result of the action rather than its cause.

It appears that the sensation of exercising free will is a poor guide in our search for the source and the time of volition. My second conclusion is that a will imposed by an independent entity such as Eccles's World 2 solves none of our problems.

At this point it looks bad for "autonomous man." Is Skinner right when he says that the existence of that creature "depends upon our ignorance," and that he "serves only to explain the things we are not yet able to explain in other ways"?[16] Must we admit then that there is no essential difference between a freely willed action and a knee jerk? Skinner demands that in a scientific approach, the "autonomous agent to which behavior has traditionally been attributed is replaced by the environment." In this approach every behavior becomes a reflex, since its outcome is determined by the environment, that is, by the stimulus. This is sometimes called the S-R approach of psychology: For every stimulus (S) there is a response (R) that must follow. Since much of the underpinning of this theory is based on animal experiments, especially experiments with rats, Koestler has contemptuously called the S-R approach the *"ratomorphic view of man."*

If we want to salvage autonomous man, we may have to do it without the help of his *sensation* of freedom, his consciousness. This means we have to divorce volition from conscious volition. If we do that, then there will no longer be an objection to having the decision-making process start a second or more before the act, as suggested in the Kornhuber experiments. It means, however, that we have to reexamine some more just what we mean by freedom. It can no longer imply an influence over the physical processes in our brains. On the contrary, autonomous man needs an autonomous brain.

Autonomy here is not isolation. The nervous system stretches, as we have seen, from sensors to effectors. It interacts continuously with the world around it. But it interacts in a way that is peculiarly and inimitably its own.

But what about the mechanistic aspects of brain function? Can they be reconciled with the concept of freedom? Determinism has always been viewed as the archenemy of freedom. Indeed, we could not ascribe freedom to a system whose dynamics is so determined that future states can be predicted precisely and far in advance. On the other hand, *some* determinism does not necessarily preclude freedom. Motivation, after all, is a form of determinism, and we would not consider it coercion if the brain leads a thirsty body to a spring. Also determinism is broken in many ways, which we will discuss in more detail in Chapter 6. In particular, the indeterminacies introduced into modern physics by quantum mechanics have often been considered a welcome relief from classical determinism. I don't believe that by itself the element of chance that appears here as a ubiquitous law of nature adds anything to one's freedom of will. It may play a part only in the hypothetical case of motivations which are so perfectly balanced that the individual finds himself on a razor's edge of indecision. This is the situation described by the medieval philosopher Buridan: A donkey stands exactly midway between two equally large and equally fragrant bales of hay and, not being able to decide which way to turn, starves to death. The tiniest push in either direction might save his life. But that is chance, not volition. What we normally understand by freedom is the *motivated* choice, not the will-o'-the-wisp of a random fluctuation.

How else can we attribute freedom of choice to the brain, a physical system however complex? I believe the answer can be found in the nature of the information flow I have sketched in Fig. 5.11 on page 171. Recall that sensory information from various receptors is relayed to the cortex, but the message contains also its own echoes, elaborated by the cortex. I stated before that the cortex is not so much a pinnacle as a hub of intersecting loops. Such a structure has enormous dynamic complexity, a feature which is completely absent in Eccles's diagram. There we find only the simple arcs from stimulus (dark arrows *up*) in Fig. 5.14, page 179, to response (white arrows *down*), and only a shadowy World 2 to rescue us from Skinnerian necessity.

This dualistic trick of overriding a mechanism by another more elusive one is shown in the picture of an endless chain of influences (Fig. 5.15 on page 181). The idea is perhaps not so absurd, nor is it entirely new. Koestler, in his book *The Ghost in the Machine*, talks about such an infinite chain of "open-ended hierarchies." Thus dualism has blossomed into pluralism. But now, I believe, we can contain this escalation, since the requisite mechanisms are all there in the physical brain. The chain of influences is there in the sensory and motor loops shown in Fig. 5.11, but instead of being open-ended it is closed upon itself, making the dynamics all the more unpredictable. If this interpretation is correct, decision making, just like perception, originates somewhere in this loop, perhaps as a minute fluctuation of neural activity. Once injected into this loop, the activity may be either amplified or squelched. If the decision is an*important one, it may involve the creation, feedback, sampling, and filtering of a multitude of images, and the schemata of simulated actions. The power of determining one's own behavior is not the power of one entity (the mind) over an-

*decided by whom or what?

other (the body), but the influence the brain has on itself, the power of self-reference. The outcome may involve elements of chance, but, more important, it will be a reflection of the unique configurations of *my* brain. In that sense my action is free.

In the more primitive example of Kornhuber's finger-bending experiments, the decisions are not of much consequence to the individual. It is my guess that, once initiated as proprioceptive schemata, they will simply be passed by the various cerebral monitors and allowed to grow in the typical explosive fashion of positive feedback. Eventually they will spill over from the somatosensory into the motor cortex and initiate the action. This may be the true meaning of the readiness potentials.

The lessons to be learned from the Kornhuber experiments concerning free will are limited by the irrelevance of the decisions made. It matters little to me whether I flex the finger now or half a second later. I value more the freedom to act in situations that have some bearing on my happiness or well-being. In that sense my will is *motivational*. It involves judging the pros and cons of alternatives before making a decision. Memories, associations, emotions, projections into the future, questions of right and wrong are involved in varying degrees.

We understand all that. What, then, *is* the problem? Our unease about the process of choosing has to do at least in part with the question whether or not we could, under the circumstances, have acted otherwise.

But there is something wrong with the question. It presupposes that the circumstances *could* be re-created in all the details, that I *could* once again be faced with the same choices. This is clearly impossible. My memory of the first instance would ensure that—even if everything else were exactly the same—I would be facing the choice under altered circumstances. We have here an example of what has been called the *contrafactual fallacy*. The re-creation of a past set of alternatives is contrafactual—against the facts as they prevail. A statement that starts with "If I had to do it over again, I would . . ." carries no more meaning than "If the moon were made of green cheese. . . ." There are many instances where the contrafactual absurdity is more evident. It makes no sense, for example, to ask *who* would be dead today if the speed limit had not been lowered to 55 mph, although it is clearly meaningful to state that so many thousands of lives have been saved by the measure.

The question of freedom of choice should not be approached by invoking the contrafactual fallacy. Instead we must content ourselves with considering our role during the decision-making process. Here we must be wary of another semantic trap. It is meaningless to portray either the "self" or "volition" as a "causal instigator." This was pointed out by the NYU neurologist Jason Brown in a thoughtful treatise entitled *Mind, Brain, and Consciousness*.[17] The self is really a "product of cognition." "Volition," says Jason Brown, "is an act of reflection that has an action as its object. Will is a way of describing the self in this reflective state."

The great commissure

"The self is a unity," Sir Charles Sherrington wrote in his classic treatise, *The Integrative Action of the Nervous System*. "It regards itself as one," he elaborates. "Others treat it as one, it is addressed as one, by a name to which it answers. The law and the state schedule it as one. It and they identify it with a body which is considered by it and them to belong to it integrally. In short, unchallenged and unargued conviction assumes it to be one. The logic of grammar endorses this by a pronoun in the singular. All its diversity is merged into oneness."[18]

How does this oneness come about, and is this still the "unchallenged and unargued conviction"?

Human features come in ones and twos. It is a curious fact that there are no triples or quadruples of anything in our bodies. But twos are the rule. All external features, and a good many of the internal ones, are bilaterally symmetrical, and most come in twos, symmetrically displaced about the midline. The few single external features have since antiquity held a special fascination, attesting, among other things, to our desire for oneness: the phallus and the navel, the traditional center of the body. In ancient Delphi a round stone was kept in the temple of Apollo. It was called the *omphalos* (Greek for navel), and was believed to mark the center of the world.

But curiously the organ of oneness, the human brain, comes in twos. A look at the old drawing by Vesalius (page 44) shows that in the relatively featureless structure of the cerebral cortex, the division between left and right *hemispheres* is the most salient aspect of the brain's anatomy. With a few exceptions, all subcortical structures are also divided into two laterally displaced, mirror symmetrical parts.

The doubleness of nervous systems is one of the oldest evolutionary

MOTOR OUTPUTS

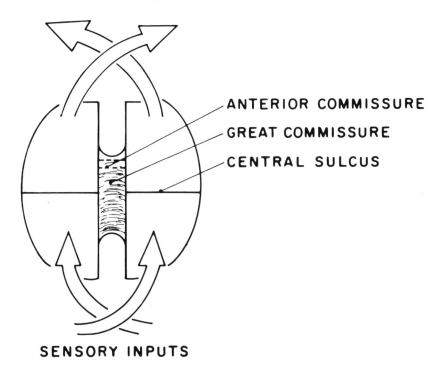

ANTERIOR COMMISSURE

GREAT COMMISSURE

CENTRAL SULCUS

SENSORY INPUTS

5.16 *The two brain hemispheres with crossed afferents and efferents, showing the great commissure, or* corpus callosum, *and its forward part, the anterior commissure*

features, going back to the bilateral bulges in the brains of *planaria* (pages 106–108). And ever since then each brain half has received sensory inputs from one side of the body, and has controlled the motor action of the same side.

In many of the invertebrates, the right brain half serves the right body half, and the left brain half the left. But somewhere during evolution, long before the arrival of vertebrates, the connections became crossed. It is not clear why and how this happened. In humans, as in all vertebrates, information from the left half of the visual field is sent to the right brain half (Fig. 4.12 on page 122), which also receives tactile and auditory stimuli from the left body half, and which controls muscles on the left side of the body.

How is unity of action achieved with this two-tracked apparatus? In the beginning the two halves were probably nearly independent. But soon the need for communication arose. When creatures changed from floating to creeping, left and right actions had to be correlated. When an object of interest, prey or predator, crossed over from one side of the visual field to the other, it was clearly of advantage to alert that part of the nervous system which was about to receive information concerning the object's progress.

At any rate, in humans the two hemispheres are interconnected by the thickest cable in the entire nervous system, the 200 million fibers of the *great commissure*, also known as the *corpus callosum*. This structure is a broad band of tissue linking the two hemispheres. We see it in the Vesalius sketch on page 44, and also in the schematic diagrams on pages 63 and 179. Figure 5.16 shows once again in diagrammatic form the crossed sensory and motor functions of the two hemispheres, and the great commissure between them. All sensory information enters the cerebral cortex somewhere behind the lateral midline, the *central sulcus*; all motor commands issue from parts forward of the central sulcus. One part of the commissure that plays a special role is a narrow cable toward the front and slightly below the main part of the corpus callosum. It is called the *anterior commissure*.

Information flows across the commissure in both directions, from left to right and from right to left. This transfer provides each hemi-

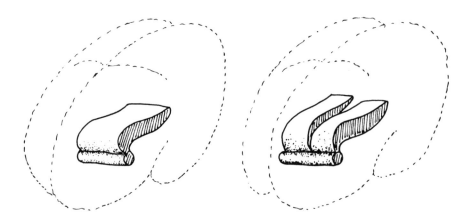

5.17 *The great commissure seen in its location in the human brain. The anterior commissure is the cylindrical tract in the lowest part of the commissure. The diagram on the right shows a "split brain" operation in which the anterior commissure was left intact.*

sphere with a complete copy of sensory information received by the other. Thus the visual cortex in the left hemisphere receives direct input (via the left LGN) from the right half of the visual field. At the same time, it is informed by the right hemisphere over the *corpus callosum* about everything that goes on in the left half of the field.

A simple experiment reported by R. Efron[19] illustrates this situation. Normal human subjects were presented with brief light flashes appearing in pairs, one in the right visual field, the other in the left visual field. The subjects were able to control the timing of the flashes until the two *appeared* to occur simultaneously. Efron found that for this to happen, the flash on the left had to occur several thousandths of a second *before* the one on the right. The explanation for this phenomenon is simply this: The left is the *dominant* hemisphere. It is also the one which is endowed with most if not all the language faculties, and it is the only one capable of speech. In the case of the experiment described here, it is clear that the judgment about the simultaneity of the two flashes is made and communicated by the left hemisphere. It receives the neural message about the flash on the right by the direct visual pathway: retina to left LGN to left visual cortex. The flash on the left side is perceived by the left hemisphere by a more circuitous route: retina to right LGN to right visual cortex to left visual cortex (through the *corpus callosum*). The true time delay measured between the two flashes, when they appear to be simultaneous, is thus the extra time it takes the message to cross the commissure from the right to the left hemisphere.

The experiment points up another important fact: The conscious judgment in this task appears to be firmly rooted in the left cerebral hemisphere. The unequal use of the two hemispheres is characteristic of the adult human brain. There is evidence, however, that in early childhood the two sides have more nearly equal faculties.[20] Language skills develop bilaterally. Only later are they taken over almost completely by the left hemisphere. Also the commissure is poorly developed in children, hence we might expect relatively little crosstalk between left and right. Children, it seems, are endowed with two rather independent brains.

If the left brain half turns out to dominate most of our decision making and our linguistic transactions, then what functions does the right hemisphere serve? This has been a topic of lively research and much speculation. The known facts come from three principal sources. The oldest is the study of deficiencies that result from injury, disease, and surgical removal of parts of the brain. A second source of information is a diagnostic technique in which one brain half or the other may be anesthetized in a way which leaves the other half awake and functioning normally. But the most startling information has come from surgery on patients with certain severe forms of epilepsy. It has been shown that severing all or part of the commissures can produce lasting relief from the severe symptoms of the disease, but brings about some important neurological and psychological changes. These have been studied in great detail by Michael Gazzaniga at Cornell University Medical College and reported in his book *The Bisected Brain*.[21]

What has emerged is that, with some exceptions, the right hemisphere is incapable of speech and hence cannot answer verbally, although it may have some linguistic comprehension and be able to spell (using letters from a Scrabble set) or even write.

But there are things the right hemisphere apparently can do better than the left. Tasks involving spatial visualization are in that category. Gazzaniga believes that these right-hemisphere specialties are functions that all have to do in one way or another with manipulative skills. Right-brain dominance in these skills is explained by the fact that the corresponding areas in the left brain half have been recruited for linguistic skills. Gazzaniga offers an interesting theory that explains why language skills have emerged in an area originally dedicated to manipulative skills. He believes the need for a language arose when man began to use tools extensively. The naming of tools then developed in the same centers that controlled the skills.

Popular articles have made much of the left-right distinctions in brain performance. The right hemisphere has been presented as the artistic side, the left as the logical one, the right described as supporting imagination and "Eastern thought," the left as plodding along in Western "linear thinking." Courses advertised in popular journals purport to teach the "balanced use" of both hemispheres. Such misinformation is deplorable. The facts are that information on left- and right-brain specialization is scarce and much of it controversial. Beyond the fact that language is, in most persons, pretty much a left-hemisphere skill, little can be said about specialization of either brain half.

The split-brain operations have produced, however, some bizarre situations and have raised some intriguing questions. When a subject is allowed to examine a small object, such as a spoon, a pencil or a coin, with his left hand, the tactile information goes to his right brain half.

With the *corpus callosum* transsected, this information cannot cross over to the left hemisphere. When the subject is asked what he had in his hand, he may answer "nothing" or "I don't know." But when he is shown a picture of many objects, the right brain half readily directs the left hand to point to the one his hand had examined. The right hemisphere has the information but cannot speak, if indeed it understands the question. The left, or speaking, hemisphere has no way of knowing.

And yet something comes across at times. The instruction to "kiss" the instructor was given to the right hemisphere of an adolescent boy with a transsected *corpus callosum*. (This can be achieved by projecting the message on the left half of a screen in front of the subject.) In this case the boy reacted with great agitation and the words "Hey, no way. You've got to be kidding." When asked what he meant, he could not explain what made him say that. The emotional content of the message apparently was transmitted, probably through the anterior commissure, which had been left intact. However, the message itself remained the secret of the right hemisphere. A young woman giggled and showed embarrassment when the picture of a naked woman was shown to her right brain half. When asked why she was laughing, she answered, "That's a funny machine," but again the speaking hemisphere was unaware of the content of the stimulus.

Such phenomena pose serious questions about the location and uniqueness of human consciousness. John Eccles, whose theory of free will we discussed in the last section, believes that only the left hemisphere has consciousness, and that the right is an automaton. But Gazzaniga reports the case of a split-brain patient whose right brain half exhibited a sense of selfhood and purpose and an unusual amount of linguistic ability. When the question "Who are you?" was posed to the right brain half, the subject was able to select letters from a Scrabble set and spell his own name: PAUL. In the same way the right brain half communicated its job preference, "car racing." But the left brain half's answer to the same question was "draftsman." We are led to conclude that the split-brain patient has not only two independently functioning brains, but also two distinct seats of consciousness. Most of the time the outsider communicates with just one of these two personalities, the left, talkative brain. When that half observes incongruous or inexplicable behavior in the body it shares with its mute companion, it will frequently invent an explanation and pretend there is no conflict (the woman who explains her embarrassed laugh by saying, "That's a funny machine"). In this way the brain attempts to reunite what has been surgically severed, to present to the outside world a false picture of unity.

Gazzaniga believes that similar processes are at work in the normal human brain, where some unifying drive continuously operates on diverse and quasi-autonomous subsystems. The unification, or appearance of unification, comes about, according to Gazzaniga, through the "verbal system." "The environment," he says, "has ways of planting hooks in our minds, and while the verbal system may not know the why or what of it all, part of its job is to make sense out of the emotional and other mental systems and, in so doing, allow man, with his mental complexity, *the illusion of a unified self.*" (My italics.)

Is the unity, then, of which Sherrington spoke so eloquently an illusion? Is it possible that our brains, which can falsify our sensations of time and place (pages 100–101), can deceive us also about that which we are most certain about: our selfhood? I quote Gazzaniga again from his very readable book, *The Integrated Mind*:

> The mind is not a psychological entity but a sociological entity, being composed of many submental systems. What can be done surgically and through hemisphere anesthetization are only exaggerated instances of a more general phenomenon. The uniqueness of man, in this regard, is his ability to verbalize and, in so doing, create a personal sense of conscious reality out of the multiple systems present.[22]

In this view our personalities are even more fragmented than McLean's creature with the *triune brain* (pages 115–116). And all these separate needs, drives, emotions, this *"sociological entity,"* is held together, if not exactly unified, by what Gazzaniga calls the *verbal system.* It is language which, like a good interpreter, mediates between the different factions and sometimes, when the interpreter doesn't understand himself, makes up a story for the sake of harmony.

Most of us would find the idea of a loosely linked multiple personality disturbing. Still, consciousness emerges in this picture as an unitary thing, tied closely to the *verbal system.* Much more disturbing is the viewpoint taken by Roland Puccetti, a philosopher at Dalhousie University in Halifax, Canada. After carefully reviewing the evidence of split-brain patients, Puccetti comes to the conclusion that the brain harbors two distinct conscious selves who are "freed by the surgery to perceive and respond independently," but are a twosome even before.

A moment's reflection will show that introspection is no help at all in either proving or dispelling this notion. *I* am, of course, the verbal self, the one who talks, and the *you* I know is also the talking, left-hemisphere you. Are there others? Perhaps I could ask my silent partner to confirm his presence by some simple gesture. "If you are there, raise *our* left arm!" Nothing happens. If the left arm goes up, it is because *I* (left-brain-half *I*) will it to do so. It is no use. My *doppelgänger*, if he exists, is used to letting *me* handle all decisions. Perhaps my other self would prefer at this moment to drive a racing car rather than help me with this book. But he dutifully directs my left hand to hold this pad of paper while the right one writes.

In the intact brain, sensory information is transferred both ways by the commissures so that each brain half has a complete picture of the world. But when the commissure is severed, the left, talking hemisphere suddenly loses sensory information about the left half of the world. It is as though a curtain had suddenly been drawn. But no split-brain patient ever complained about that loss. "One would miss the departure of a good friend more, apparently," says Gazzaniga, "than the left hemisphere misses the right." Nor has the right hemisphere, after being released from bondage by the surgeon's knife, ever conveyed to anyone a memory of its servitude and domination by the left. Perhaps that is because no one has yet asked the right question. Perhaps both of these are instances of what Puccetti calls "the integrative drive of the cortex, the compulsion to deny at all costs the presence in the same cranium of that congenital aphasic who sometimes survives us after massive left-sided lesions."

Consciousness: What is it? Where is it? Who has it? Why?

If the myth is tragic, that is because the hero is conscious.
—A. CAMUS, *The Myth of Sisyphus*

We have come a long way since John Watson's bold assertion that "the time has come when psychology must discard all reference to consciousness," and that "introspection can play no part" in our description of brain function. Most psychologists today would deem their science severely impoverished if they had to heed Watson's advice.

Consider the following facts: A great variety of sense organs collect information about the outside world as well as about internal conditions of our body, and convey this information to the central nervous system. I am able to report on *some* of that information. I can tell you what appears in my field of vision, what sounds my ears pick up, and the feel of an object I touch. But if you were to ask me about the level of the enzyme gastrin in my stomach or about the acidity of my blood, I could not answer you. This information is recorded by sensors and *used* by the central nervous system in important regulatory functions. But that speaking and reporting entity we sometimes call the "conscious self" knows nothing about these facts. It is as though they had gone to another brain not connected with mine.

It requires no further definition to say that I am *conscious* of visual, auditory, tactile, and many other types of sensory information, and that I am *unconscious* of others. We have discussed the startling phenomenon of *blindsight* (page 127), in which subjects with surgically removed visual cortices can nevertheless perform discrimination tasks in the "blind" region of the visual field. At the same time, they deny having any *sensation* of light in that region.

These examples show most strikingly that a clear distinction can be made between sensory messages that enter my consciousness and those which don't. Only the first kind I call *sensations*.

My knowledge of sensations is most direct. I call it *introspection*, which is something of a misnomer. I don't have to *direct my gaze inward*, as the term suggests. Having a sensation is not an *action*, though it is often the result of an action. Nobody has to define sensations for me. Nobody *can* define them for me. They are the only certainty I have. They are the elementary building blocks, the *quarks* of my philosophy.

I assume that you, too, have sensations. This assumption or *axiom* I base on my observation of your behavior as well as on my knowledge of our close biological kinship. You and I not only look alike outside *and* under our skin. Our genes have faced the same world for millions of years and dealt with it in very similar ways. I find it easy, therefore, to believe that you, too, feel happy when you laugh. It is an assumption I find most persuasive, but it cannot be derived from any compelling rules of logic.

The biological kinship is also the reason why I attribute sensation not only to other humans but also to animals, especially the higher forms. This axiom forms the cornerstone of a system of ethics that binds together all living things. (Of course, all my interpersonal relationships and practically all my endeavors were based on the validity of this assumption long before I came to formalize its axiomatic nature.)

I do not feel compelled to attribute sensations to a machine, though I could do so if I wanted to. A robot may show the right behavior, but I choose not to believe it when it says it feels a pain. Part of the reason is the profound difference between its heritage and mine. The lovable, affectionate computer of science-fiction movies is the result of an extrapolation that attaches undue significance to behavioral similarity and overlooks our essential difference in kind.

The attribution of sensation and thought to *all* inanimate objects, as proposed by the school of panpsychism, lacks even the support of a behavioral similarity. The same is true for a consciousness that is not attached to a thing, living or inanimate, as in some Eastern philosophies. William James says, "My thought belongs with my other thoughts, and your thought belongs with your other thoughts. Whether anywhere in the room there be a mere thought, which is nobody's thought, we have no means of ascertaining." He goes on to say that "the only states of consciousness that we naturally deal with are found in personal consciousness, minds . . ." I would go a step farther and say that we know of no consciousness that is not based in a brain.

Sensations are brought about by our senses. They involve all the complicated neural mechanisms of which we spoke in Chapter 4, and many more still to be discovered. But none of these processes can *explain* the phenomenon of sensation. It has been called an *epiphenomenon*, or an *emerging quality*—something that appears at a certain level of complexity. This explains little but tends to suggest that if I were only to duplicate the complexity in a machine, I would have created consciousness.

I have used *sensation* and *consciousness* almost synonymously. To have a sensation is to be conscious. A "conscious sensation" is therefore a redundancy. The range of sensations of which an animal is capable and the repertory of its consciousness are probably very nearly the same. But with humans something new enters the picture: language. Consider this situation: Two persons are sitting in a room, and one says to the other, "Have you noticed that it is getting cold in here?" The other has felt the cold also—that is, he was conscious of it—but his thoughts had been occupied with other things. He answers something like, "Yes, now that you mention it."

While he had the sensation of cold all along, he is now also observing, sensing his own verbalization of the fact that he felt cold. His attention is now preoccupied with the subject, and he may say, aloud or to himself, "There must be an open window," or "Something must be wrong with the furnace." We see here the expansion of conscious activity that results from what Gazzaniga has called the *verbal system*.

Earlier in this section we spoke about a "sketchpad in the head" which would allow us to *simulate* the occurrence of events, and we theorized that such *thoughts* might produce afferent neural activity that in some way resembles sensory inputs. If this picture is correct, then the sensations resulting from such simulated inputs are also part of our consciousness. It is thus possible to take away the external stimulus of cold and *think* about the cold that may come months from now, or conjure up the sensations of a freezing day last winter. This, too, relies—at least in part—on our use of the *verbal system*.

On the other hand, I believe it is going much too far to assert that no consciousness can exist without a verbal system. Such a view would deny consciousness to all animals except humans and would degrade the status of sensations. It can be shown in fact that events can be simulated, or thought about, without recourse to language.

Let us do a simple experiment. Take a piece of paper and a pencil or pen. Now write your signature. The act, if you carried it out, was accompanied by a number of sensations. There was the feel of pressure against your fingertips. There were sensations from your skin and joints as your hand rapidly shifted position, and you heard the sound of the writing tip gliding over the paper. Your eyes meanwhile observed your moving hand and the familiar line pattern being formed on the paper. Now, put the paper and your writing utensil aside and *think* through the same action. Try not to move your wrist or even tense your muscles. You can go through the entire act in "real time," and know exactly where you are at any moment.

Some of you may have done just what I asked you to do. But I suspect that the majority never did pick up the pencil and paper. Knowing exactly what would happen, you simulated the action the first time. But this only demonstrates one of the many ways in which we use simulated or synthetic action in place of the real thing. You may say that writing one's name certainly involves a verbal system. But I could have asked you also to think of a tennis serve or strumming a guitar. Since this does not, in my opinion, necessitate any use of language, there is no reason to doubt that animals, too, have and use this faculty of simulating events. It is not unlikely that the hawk, before he swoops down on his prey, or the tiger before he leaps, has a "mental image" of the act and uses that to check his progress.

It appears, however, that our use of simulated action is far more extensive than that of any animal. A dog that has become entangled with his chain is often unable to extricate himself. A look at his situation tells me that if he walked clockwise around the tree he would be free. Apparently the dog's brain is unable to form a clear image of its own dilemma and "see" its way out.

The advanced ability to solve problems by simulated acts is perhaps man's greatest intellectual asset. The emergence of tools is, I believe, not so much the result of fortuitous "puttering," as of his ability to scan mentally a great variety of shapes and to sample their uses before actually making them.

The *where* of consciousness has been as elusive as the *how*. The strong involvement of language faculties would implicate the cerebral cortex. Of course, this is also where all sensory inputs terminate. But Wilder Penfield, after many years of carrying out brain surgery, came to the conclusion that no one part of the cortex can be singled out as the seat of, or even as essential to, consciousness. On the other hand, it *is* necessary that the cortex be *aroused* by signals from a part of the brainstem called the reticular activating system (RAS). Again, as discussed in the beginning of Chapter 4, I favor a position which views the cortex as only a link between more peripheral structures on the afferent and efferent sides. This hypothesis would also explain why activity in one part of the cortex produces one sensation, say of a sound, while similar activity in a different location may mean light or touch. The cortex, remember, has remarkably similar structure in all these sensory areas. This again suggests that cortical activity mediates between specific fiber systems, and that consciousness, rather than residing in a particular cortical location, is a property of a larger system which includes some of the peripherals.

In Chapter 4 (page 100) I briefly referred to a set of experiments reported by Benjamin Libet, a neurophysiologist at the University of California collaborating with the neurosurgeon Bertram Feinstein at the Mt. Zion Neurological Institute in San Francisco.[23] Libet is concerned with the timing of the conscious response to a stimulus. He emphasizes that the instant at which a subject is able to respond to a stimulus by an action of his own is not necessarily the time at which he becomes conscious of the event. Consciousness, he maintains, can be ascertained only by introspection. The outsider must rely on a verbal report by the subject. Accordingly, Libet's experiments are performed on humans who are undergoing or have undergone brain surgery in which wire electrodes have been implanted in their brains for therapeutic purposes, and who have consented to certain tests being performed.

Libet has concentrated his efforts on sensations of stimuli applied to the skin or to corresponding regions in the somatosensory pathway. This sensory system goes from receptors in the skin via fibers in the spinal cord and relay nuclei in the brainstem and thalamus to the somatosensory cortex, the region just behind the central sulcus (Fig.4.21 on page 141). He has succeeded in applying electrical stimuli directly to the somatosensory cortex in such a way that the patient has a sensation similar to that elicited by a natural stimulus, for example, by pressure being applied at some point on the skin. It was found, though, that this cortical stimulation must be sustained for a minimum length of time, depending somewhat on the stimulus strength. Any stimulation shorter than that minimum was not reported by the patient. It produced no conscious response. The minimum stimulus duration necessary for a conscious response was, for low intensities, about half a second. Similar results were obtained when the electrical signal was applied to the thalamic relay nucleus rather than to the cortex.

By contrast, Libet found that very brief stimuli applied to the skin at the weakest effective strength always led to sensation. Even a single action potential produced on the periphery could be accompanied by a conscious response. Perhaps, he thought, these peripheral stimuli are recognized by the brain more readily as the *real thing*, and therefore require only a short duration before the conscious response sets in. He soon found, however, that when an electrical stimulus was applied to the somatosensory cortex some 0.2 seconds or more *after* the skin stimulus, the subject failed to be conscious of the skin stimulus. It follows that again several tenths of a second must elapse between the signal and conscious response. This is more than ten times as long as it takes the skin stimulus to reach the cortex. The cortical stimulus thus appears to reach back in time and erase the record of the earlier skin stimulus. This effect is known as *backward masking*. The sequence of events is shown graphically in Fig. 5.18. A strong stimulus is able to *mask*, that is, prevent the conscious recognition of an earlier event. The assumption is that such an erasure can take place only before the first event has entered consciousness. On this assumption, the longest

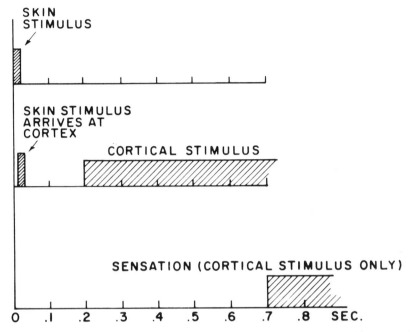

5.18 *Backward masking. A cortical stimulus following about 2/10 second after a skin stimulus* masks *the skin stimulus. The subject is conscious only of the cortical stimulus.*

time interval that produces backward masking is the minimum time it takes for a stimulus to reach consciousness. The conclusion is therefore that several tenths of a second must elapse between stimulus and sensation, whether the stimulus is *real*,—applied to the skin—or intro-duced at the cortex.

The next experiment came therefore as something of a surprise. Libet sought to establish the true timing of a sensation. It would seem that the most direct way to go about this would be to have the subject give a quick signal (snapping a finger, pushing a button) as soon as he senses the stimulus. But this would show only that the neural information was received and "processed," not that a conscious response was achieved. A more roundabout method is thus needed. Libet used two stimuli, one to the skin and one to the cortex. The subject could readily distinguish between the two and was asked which of the two *sensations* occurred first. The timing of the stimuli is shown in Fig. 5.19: The cortical stimulus starts first and is followed several tenths of a second later by the skin stimulus. The cortical stimulus causes a conscious

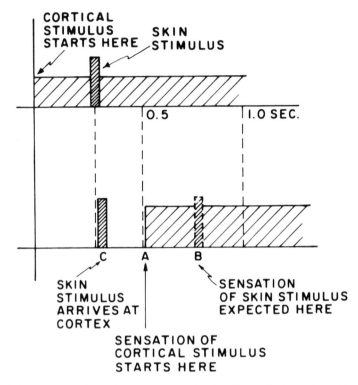

CORTICAL
STIMULUS
STARTS HERE

SKIN
STIMULUS

0.5

1.0 SEC.

C

A

B

SKIN
STIMULUS
ARRIVES AT
CORTEX

SENSATION
OF SKIN STIMULUS
EXPECTED HERE

SENSATION OF
CORTICAL STIMULUS
STARTS HERE

5.19 *Subjective timing of sensations of stimuli applied to the skin and to the somatosensory cortex. (After Benjamin Libet)*

response about half a second after it starts, that is, at point A in the diagram. The skin stimulus takes a short time to arrive at the cortex (about ten to twenty thousandths of a second), and should reach consciousness about half a second after that (point B in Fig. 5.19). However, the subject reports that the skin sensation came *before* the sensation of the cortical stimulus. Thus, although the backward masking and other data strongly suggest that about half a second elapses in both cases before a conscious response is produced, the subjective timing is *referred* in the second case to an instant close to the actual event, or point C.

Libet furnishes an explanation for this phenomenon. When an electrode is used to record the electric potential on the brain surface following a stimulus to the skin, the observed time course looks somewhat like the curve shown in Fig. 5.20. This is actually an average taken over many trials and is called the *averaged evoked response,* or

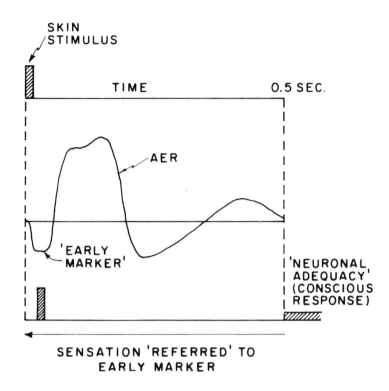

5.20 *Skin stimulus, average evoked response (AER), and conscious response. (After Benjamin Libet)*

AER. The AER has an "early" component, the sharp surface positive swing that occurs immediately after the stimulus. It is followed by slower negative and positive waves, which extend out to and beyond the time Libet found "adequate" for eliciting conscious response (about one half second). Libet calls this "neuronal adequacy." Nevertheless, the subjective judgment of the timing places sensation of the event much earlier, about the time of the early component of the AER. Libet believes that this part of the AER acts as a time *marker* to which the sensation *will* be referred, if and when the neural activity reaches the adequate timing, half a second later. Since the characteristic time marker of the early AER is absent in the case of cortical stimulation, the referral of the sensation backward in time cannot take place.

I will summarize briefly these most peculiar findings: A conscious response to a stimulus cannot occur, according to Libet, unless some form of neuronal reverberation continues for up to about half a second, the *adequate* time for sensation. On the other hand, *when* sensation sets in, the subjective judgment of its timing *refers* it back close to the time when the actual event took place. It appears that sensations are replays of events that are well in the past, but manage to convey to us the delusion of a conscious immediacy and participation.

Assuming all this is right, are we then the victims of a grandiose hoax? The answer lies, I believe, in the fact that the significance of an event (for us) does not end with the event. What it can teach us continues long after the sensation has departed, but only if there *had been* a sensation. Erwin Schrödinger, in his essay "Mind and Matter,"[24] calls consciousness "the tutor who supervises the education of the living substance." Thus my actions now may not be caused by my present conscious participation, but they are certainly guided by what I felt and thought in the past. Besides, I have at my disposal a verbal system which not only facilitates my access to past events but also helps me to compile, correlate, and evaluate the past, and to project, simulate, and sample the future. With all this in my consciousness, the loss of half a second out of the present does not seem so distressing.

6

THIS UNCERTAIN
WORLD

*There lives more faith in honest doubt, Believe me, than in half
the creeds.*

—ALFRED LORD TENNYSON

I have led you through discussions on brain structure, brain development, the physiology of vision, the functioning of whole brains and
half brains. Now I am about to take you on a detour through territory
that includes physics, mathematics, and even a bit of cosmology. What
for? you may ask. I feel a little like an Alpine guide who urges his
client over yet another tiresome obstacle, with only the promise that
the view will be better on the other side.

That physics should have anything to tell us about mind may come
as a surprise. Physicists have traditionally stressed the objective qualities of the universe, that is, those which, upon measurement, yield the
same values for *any* observer. This has been taken as an indication
that the measurements were in fact independent of the observer, or
objective. But modern physics has forced us into dilemmas in which
we find it difficult, if not impossible, to maintain the neat separation
between the observer and the observed. The human observing any part
of nature becomes part of the dynamics of what he observes. This is
not just due to the physical procedures he employs in his measurements. Even his prior knowledge affects the state of the physical system he examines. There has been a significant shift from Eddington's

view, which regarded life as an insignificant and very local accident in the universe, to that of John Wheeler, who speaks of the "universe of mind and man." This shift is to a large extent the result of that part of modern physics we call *quantum mechanics*. Contemporary physicists have expressed the view that just as mind and consciousness enter into questions about the universe at large, so the findings of modern physics have something to tell us about the human mind.

I will begin this part of the book with a discussion of the large and the small in physics, and the classical treatments of these two worlds. I want to show here that *chaos*, that is, *unpredictability*, invades many macroscopic processes, even in what is known as the *classical regime*. I believe this fact to be significant when we consider the dynamics of brain function. The picture is further and severely complicated by the character of self-reference, which we have mentioned a few times before, and finally by quantum mechanics. I hope that these discussions, if they do not improve the vistas, will at least dispel the notion still held by many biologists that the laws of physics, if only cleverly and diligently applied, will ultimately reveal the absolute determinism and predictability in any physical process, however complex.

The scales of things

Sizes in the physical universe range from those of the subnuclear entities, like the elusive *quarks*, to that of the universe itself—a vast, expanding sphere containing many billions of galaxies. The scale of time intervals a physicist must contemplate is equally enormous, from the shortest lifetimes of some of the *elementary particles* (less than one billionth of a trillionth of a second) to the present age of the universe, some fifteen billion years, and beyond.

Occupying minute intervals on both of these scales are the things that are of immediate concern to humans—sizes of objects that we can hold or examine directly, that are comparable to our own stature, and times not too different from the ones that punctuate our lives—the span of a breath or a life.

It is not surprising that physics began as a study of events on these *human* scales. Galileo Galilei began this endeavor in the late sixteenth and early seventeenth century by carefully observing the swings of pendulums and the falling of objects. But he soon extended his observations to objects on an astronomical scale. Galileo discovered the moons of the planet Jupiter and their motions, and Sir Isaac Newton —born in 1642, the year Galileo died—formulated the law governing the first universal force, that of gravity. He deduced this law from observations of planets circling the sun. It is a law of startling simplicity, and it predicts with enormous precision the falling of an apple from a tree, the movements of moons around planets, of planets around the sun, of stars around galactic centers, and many other phenomena over vastly different scales.

The gravitational force is but *one* of the universal forces. There are four that are recognized and studied by modern physicists, and, curiously, gravitation is the weakest of them all. The others are the *electromagnetic forces,* the *strong forces,* and the *weak forces.*

Very roughly speaking, each of these four forces defines a *realm,* or range of scales, in the universe. The gravitational forces, as we have seen already, play a significant role in the dynamics of objects from apples to galaxies. Electromagnetic forces operate in general on a smaller scale. Although we can demonstrate and use electric phenomena on a household scale (light bulbs, radios, etc.), their true realm is at the level of atoms and molecules. The different particles making up these structures (atomic nuclei and electrons) are held together almost exclusively by electromagnetic forces. Gravitational forces between them exist, as between all masses in the universe, but they are so minute as to be negligible.

When we go down into the world of atomic nuclei, we find particles like *protons* and *neutrons,* and also what has been called a "zoo" of critters, a baffling variety of unstable particles, the *mesons.* In this realm the strong force, the third universal force, dominates the action, with electromagnetic forces playing a minor role and gravitational forces again completely negligible. Finally, the weak forces come into play as some of these subnuclear particles change into others: neutrons into protons, mesons into other mesons or into other lighter particles.

I mention all this to bring out one important point: While the *realms* of which we spoke do not have absolutely sharp boundaries, we can nevertheless make some significant and practical separations. A proton in the nucleus of a helium atom cares little about whether the atom is part of a liquid at −453 degrees Fahrenheit, or a hot gas streaming out of the mouth of a volcano, or trapped in the hot interior of a star. On a more classical and down-to-earth scale, the physics of Galileo and Newton treats objects almost as inviolate entities: A pendulum bob is a small, massive object of precise location and precisely predictable motion. Atoms, of course, were not discovered until much later, but Newton was firmly convinced of the atomistic nature of things, a point of view inherited from ancient Greek philosophers. Still, he treated the dynamics of objects as though such internal structure, and perhaps internal motion, of the parts could safely be disregarded when considering the gross motions of the swinging pendulum or the orbiting planets. The wonder of it is that this convenient overlooking of detail—Newton could not have done otherwise—led to a mechanics so rigorous and so successful that faith in the absolute predictability of events dominated physics for the next two and a half centuries.

The atomistic nature of matter was confirmed, and it was not long before atoms and molecules, though unseen, became household words. It soon became evident also that they were in continuous motion, exerted forces on each other, and occasionally bounced off one another like billiard balls. There was at first no question that they would have to observe the same laws of mechanics that Galileo and Newton had derived for larger objects. There was, however, the difficulty of direct observation and the further complication that molecules, unlike billiard balls, could not readily be studied one or two at a time, because they usually occurred in vast numbers. There are about twenty billion molecules in a thimbleful of air.

If we wanted to know what happens to this thimbleful of air, it would be a hopeless task to localize each molecule and determine precisely how its motion is affected by the presence of all the other molecules. Instead a method called *statistical mechanics* is used, in which it is assumed that the molecules are randomly distributed, have certain average speeds and certain probabilities of colliding with one another. This allows us to describe what is known as the *macrostate* of the system. It tells us something about the gross aspects of the substance, but not where each molecule is located or how it is moving. If we knew all that, we would know the *microstate* of the system. In general, macrostates are readily determined by observation, microstates are not.

The question is often asked whether we could overcome our ignorance concerning the microstate of a system. Why can't we *in principle*, and eventually perhaps *in practice*, for a small amount of carefully isolated matter determine the positions and velocities of every molecule at a given instant? Then, using the laws of mechanics, we might calculate the precise *trajectories* and find out what molecule will collide with what other molecule, at what instant and at what location. In this way we should be able to ascertain the precise state, that is, the *microstate* of this system for any future time.

The answer to the above question is simply that it cannot be done. For reasons that are somewhat technical, the microstate of a macroscopic system cannot be determined. But even if we *could* determine it, it would be of little use to us. We would need almost infinite precision in our measurements to compute only a little way into the future. Even this would require a computer of monumental proportions. However, soon—in something like a millionth of a second—we would lose all knowledge of the microstate because of minute influences from outside that can neither be measured nor controlled. It was calculated that the movement of a few pounds of material at the distance of our nearest star, Alpha Centauri, light years away, would be sufficient to shake up our carefully determined microstate beyond all hope of recovery.

The microworld is thus inherently *chaotic*. A small bit of matter, just visible under the microscope and suspended in a gas, is seen to go through jerky, completely unpredictable motions that result from the random agitation of the gas molecules.

That the macroscopic world nevertheless often appears ordered and predictable is a result of the great separation in scale. The pen I am holding as I write this is made up of an enormous number of molecules. My ignorance concerning the state of any of these is *averaged out*, made irrelevant by their sheer number: The pen does not wriggle but rests obediently in my hand. Our faith in the scientific predictability of events is the result of this vast gap between microscopic and macroscopic events. We will see in the next section, however, that there may be cross talk between the two realms. When this happens, microscopic uncertainty can be injected into the macroscopic world.

In the chaotic realm of atoms and molecules, there exist structures which appear to be anomalies, almost paradoxes: the minute structures that make up the most elementary subsystems of living organisms. We find here complicated assemblies of molecules with highly precise and stable configurations. The DNA molecule and its associated protein molecules are the guardians of detailed genetic information that must be preserved with great precision for many years and at the relatively high body temperature of 98 degrees Fahrenheit. How such molecular order can persist in the chaotic molecular world is a problem that was discussed by Erwin Schrödinger in his classic book

What Is Life?[1] The paradox can be explained only by *quantum mechanics,* which replaces Newtonian mechanics on the microscopic scale. Schrödinger himself was one of the founders of quantum mechanics.

In the human brain the range of scales extends from gross structures (cortex, cerebellum, etc.) down to the world of atoms and molecules. At the lowest end are the chaotic *thermal* motions but also some remarkably stable molecular mechanisms, such as the action of transmitter molecules at the synapses. At intermediate levels there are the vast numbers of individual cells, the neurons, and, near the top, the readily distinguishable neural masses and pathways. The trouble is we don't really know where within this wide range the significant action takes place. It has been tacitly assumed by most physiologists that what ultimately counts is just the firing of the neurons. But is it the firing of *every* neuron? If so, then we have a system of immense complexity, and we must ask ourselves again whether it is, in principle, possible to determine at any time the complete state of the system, and to what extent the dynamics can be computed.

Chaos in the cosmos

Life on earth owes its existence to the relatively stable conditions that have prevailed here for the last few billion years: a nearby star—our sun—whose brilliance has not changed significantly in all this time, and a planet—our home—that has kept its respectable distance from the sun, never coming too close to its searing heat and never venturing too far out into the cold depths of outer space. We take for granted the stability of the earth's near-circular orbit around the sun. It has been repeated with very minor variations several billion times.

If we have come to expect this kind of stability and predictability in other physical systems as well, this is probably due to the fact that physicists have in the past concentrated their efforts on systems with "well-behaved" dynamics. Orbits of stars, planets, moons, satellites, and missiles have been calculated with great precision, but nobody has even tried to compute the trajectories of tumbling dice. There is a simple reason: It can't be done, so not much was said about it.

But recently physicists have gone back to classical mechanics for another look at the intractables: the so-called *chaotic systems.*

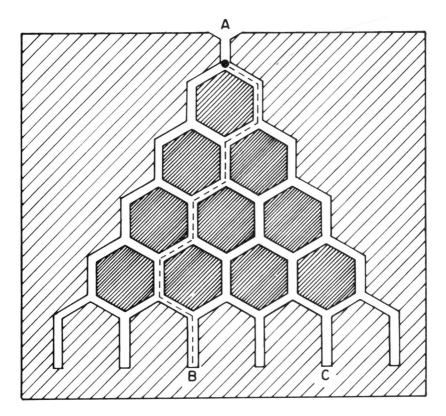

6.1 *A game of chance. The ball dropped in at the top of the maze will arrive in one of the six bins at the bottom. The outcome of any one trial cannot be predicted with certainty.*

A simple illustration will show what is involved. Figure 6.1 is a diagram of a game of chance, a variation of which is the pinball machine. A ball enters at the top of the maze and falls on a succession of knife-edges. Each time it hits it will have a fifty-fifty chance of dropping on one side or the other of the knife-edge. Take the case in which a ball enters at point A, follows the dotted line, and emerges at point B. Its path, or *trajectory*, should be uniquely determined by the *initial state*, that is, the precise way it entered at point A. Assume this to be true and ask how much that initial state would have to be changed in order to make the ball come out at point C instead of point B. The answer is that the two initial states are so close that they are indistinguishable from one another. The slightest shift in the beginning or anywhere along the path would make the outcome totally unpredictable. These shifts may be so small as to be neither measurable nor controllable.

Such examples used to be thought of as curiosities. However, it is becoming more apparent that *chaotic systems* are the rule rather than the exception in nature. They all have this in common: They are ordinary mechanical systems in the classical sense, but the dynamics are continually poised on knife-edge decisions whose outcome cannot be predicted. The amplification of minute errors or uncertainties often reaches factors of a trillion or more.

Perhaps the best-known and most studied example of chaotic motion is the *turbulence* observed in the flow of liquids and gases. We are familiar with the appearance of turbulence. Turn on a water faucet, at first only very slightly. You will see a smooth stream of water, its motion very regular and predictable. It looks the same from one moment to the next. This is called *laminar flow*. Now open the faucet wider, and soon, abruptly, the picture will change. Water tumbles out in irregular patterns. If you were to take flash pictures of the stream, no two pictures would be alike, and if a physicist were to take precise measurements of the exact shape of the water column at one instant, and of all other factors that may affect the flow, he would still be unable to predict the shape an instant later. The system is *chaotic*.

Having accepted the explanation that in chaotic systems minute fluctuations become rapidly amplified, we ask how do these fluctuations come about? Where is that rich invisible source of variety and change in the solid setup of the game of chance in Fig. 6.1, or the seemingly unchanging preconditions in turbulent flow?

The answer is that the microworld of ceaselessly moving molecules provides fluctuations which, in the case of the very delicately poised chaotic systems, are sufficient to intrude on the world of large-scale phenomena. The separation between the behavior of a readily observable "object," on the one hand, and the *thermal* motion of its molecules, on the other, could be maintained successfully in the case of falling apples, orbiting planets, and many other textbook examples of Newtonian dynamics. In the case of chaotic systems, this separation breaks down. In the last section we saw that we are barred from ever having detailed knowledge of the state of the microworld. It follows that our ignorance must now extend into the macroworld as well.

This problem was discussed recently by Robert Shaw,[2] a physicist at the University of California at Santa Cruz, from the point of view of information theory. Shaw pictures the production of macroscopic features in turbulence as the *flow of information* from the microworld into the macroworld. At the same time, energy flows the other way as macroscopic features are dissipated and their energies go into heat (Fig. 6.2).

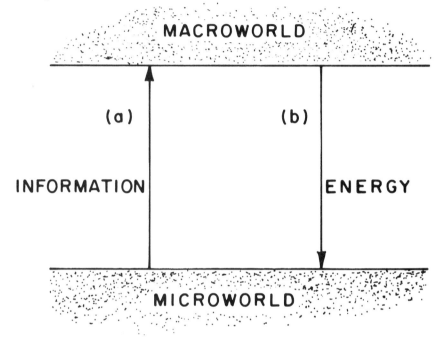

6.2 *Information flow in turbulence. (a) Generation of turbulence by thermal fluctuations; (b) dissipation; information is lost to the macroworld. (After Robert Shaw)*

I mention all this because there is a good possibility that the neural network with its ten billion interacting neurons has some of the characteristics of a chaotic system. It would be difficult to prove this, but there are hints that more than suggest the possibility. The macroscopic behavior of the brain, as observed for example in the electroencephalogram (EEG), shows a richness of form and an unpredictability that is reminiscent of turbulent flow. True, there are rhythms, that is, dominant frequencies, especially in the EEG of an inattentive subject (bottom of Fig. 6.3). Here the so-called *alpha rhythm* dominates the picture. But even in this case there is massive and wholly unpredictable detail.

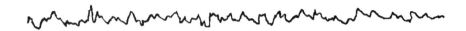

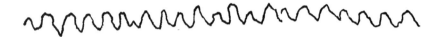

6.3 *Two EEG traces. Above: an awake, attentive subject. Below: the same subject in a state of inattention.*

A similarly chaotic picture is obtained when we look at the record of activity of a single neuron. Frequencies may rise and fall with the passage of sensory or motor messages. But the precise pattern of action potentials has never been shown to be causally related to the details of a stimulus. The spontaneous neural activity which exists in the absence of specific messages has all the characteristics of a random sequence of pulses.

If we conclude from this that the brain is a chaotic system, does this mean that neural activity is dominated by the meaningless vagaries of thermal noise? We know that this cannot be so. Our perceptions, our thoughts and actions are not random.

The explanation lies, I believe, in the existence of structural and functional levels in the brain that occupy intermediate positions within the range of scales which stretches from the molecular level to the level of observable manifestations of brain function, such as the EEG or motor action. I am thinking again of the scale of neurons. If I wanted to specify the level of excitation of each neuron and tell you which ones are firing at this instant, I would find it impossible for reasons very similar to those cited in the preceding section. There is no practical way of obtaining such a detailed picture of brain activity. Yet we are talking here about phenomena (action potentials, postsynaptic potentials) that are reasonably far above those caused by single molecules.

We find important intermediate realms also in structure. The details of neural connectivity, including numbers, distribution, and strengths of synapses, are features far above the molecular level, but also far below the level of such macroscopic structures as sensory relay nuclei, the visual cortex, the *corpus callosum*, and others. Again, while we may be able to look at a few axon trees and synaptic junctions, the complete description of the human neural network appears to be beyond experimental reach.

Memory engrams are laid down on the delicate structure of the neural network in ways we do not yet fully understand. These changes are extremely subtle and diffuse, but almost certainly supramolecular. The strengths of these engrams seem to vary over a wide range, from barely more than noise to dominating and indelible.

If we let the word "microstate" denote, as before, the precise disposition and motion of all molecules, and if by "macrostate," we mean a description of practically observable parameters (EEG or behavior, for example), then we will need another term to refer to these intermediate levels of structure and function. Let us call them *"ministates."*

Suppose now that neural dynamics is chaotic but not so chaotic as to be affected by the truly meaningless thermal fluctuations of individual molecules. Instead it is sensitive to the ministates of millions of diffuse engrams that have accumulated. If this is a correct description, then we can view thought processes as resembling a turbulent flow of information from the ministates into macroscopic neurodynamics (Fig. 6.4). At the same time, as the gross features of sensory stimuli subside, information descends into the ministates, analogous to the dissipation of macroscopic features in turbulence.

There is one significant difference, however, between the information flow in chaotic systems as described by Shaw and the information exchange I envision between macro- and ministates in the brain. When a turbulent feature subsides into thermal noise, it is irretrievably lost. Thermal motion has no memory, carries no labels. But when information is deposited into the ministates, they will retain meaning, at least for the individual, for as long as the neural machinery linking them with the macrostates remains intact. We must assume, of course, that the ministates are by and large immune to disturbances by random molecular motion. But some "leakage" of thermal noise into the macroscopic world of action cannot be ruled out (dotted arrow in Fig. 6.4). This diagram also brings out the fact that here is another loop: The upward flow of information from the cerebral ministates will give rise to the reactivation and reinforcement of the same or associated engrams, accounting both for the intensification and the progression of thought.

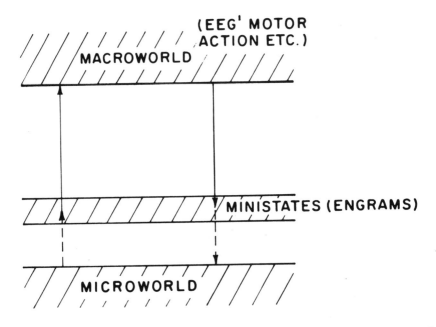

6.4 *Turbulence model of brain function. Arrows indicate the direction of the information flow. (Compare with Shaw's diagram of turbulence, Fig. 6.2)*

Self-reference *ad nauseam*

I write this chapter with some hesitation because Douglas Hofstadter, a professor of computer science at Indiana University, has recently published a marvelous and rather monumental book entitled *Gödel, Escher, Bach,*[3] which is devoted almost exclusively to the topic of self-reference. I cannot hope to come close to reaching the breadth and excitement that are conveyed in Hofstadter's work, but I feel that a brief treatment of the topic is needed in my panorama of mind and brain.

I started this chapter, appropriately, with a self-reference. The sentence beginning "I write this chapter" is in fact part of the chapter, and I am now compounding the problem by commenting on my remark concerning the writing of this chapter, all of which is still part of it. My present activity of writing, reporting on my writing, and commenting on my reporting have all become the subject matter of the book (which I am writing).

Logicians once cautioned that we must avoid all such examples of self-reference because they lead to paradoxes. A classic example is that of Epimenides, the Cretan philosopher, who said, "All Cretans are liars." (He is evidently a liar, if he spoke the truth.) Then there is the barber who shaves every man in his town except those who shave themselves (if he shaves himself, then he doesn't shave himself.)

The prescription for purging our language, our logic, and our mathematics of the troublesome contradictions and paradoxes that arise from self-referent, or *recursive,* statements was laid down in a heroic salvage attempt by Bertrand Russell and A.N. Whitehead when they published *Principia Mathematica.*[4] Then in 1931 the Austrian mathematician Kurt Gödel showed that this effort had failed, and that any similar attempt at constructing a mathematical system that was complete and free of self-referent complications must likewise fail.

The feature that causes all the complications in mathematical logic and in the functioning of the brain is the existence of loops. Some loops are straightforward. The algorithm we all use when we divide one number by another (assuming you did not grow up in the age of pocket calculators and never learned the art) takes us repeatedly around a loop by way of residues and partial answers. We stop when the residue becomes zero, or when we feel the answer is close enough. There is nothing mysterious or subtle about the procedure.

However, not all loops are of this harmless variety. Hofstadter speaks of "strange loops," in which there exists an element of surprise as you follow the loop. Often there is something disquieting or paradoxical. Strange loops sometimes leave the observer in a state of suspense or uncertainty, or just plain lost. *As in Escher's drawings*

I have stressed repeatedly that the human brain contains a number of structural loops, and that sensory messages are modified by the effects they produce at another level. The brain is the epitome of a self-referent system. My self is forever imaging itself and changing in response to the image. It can never quite catch up with itself. To this extent is also remains undefined.

The imaging process can also put me in the place of another person and allow me to observe myself from *his* vantage point and modify my own actions according to what I see. The poker player uses this device to advantage. The self-referent loop in this case is not a direct one, but comes back to me only after involving another person. The fact that the other person is also a thinking and projecting being leads to some interesting and often strange loops. Such interactions, especially those in which the participants are adversaries, have been studied in a branch of applied mathematics called *game theory*. I will give some examples from a book by Vladimir Lefebvre called *The Structure of Awareness*.[5] First, here is a simple situation in which the participants have the same, nonconflicting interests.

A prisoner is kept in a jail which has an irregular polygonal shape, shown in Fig. 6.5. He hopes to escape with the aid of an accomplice

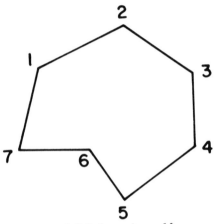

6.5 *Prisoner's problem*

outside. To do this, he and his accomplice must dig from opposite ends at one of the seven corners of the jail. They can succeed only if they choose the same corner. No communication is possible between the prisoner and his accomplice. For a second put yourself in the position of the prisoner (or his accomplice) and decide at what corner you are going to dig. The chances are that you will choose corner 6 because it is *different* from all the others. This in itself does not make it better, but you guess correctly that the man on the other side of the wall will make the same choice. *His* only motivation for doing so, however, is *his* guess that *you* might do so. Thus, although neither the prisoner nor his accomplice sees any intrinsic advantage in picking corner 6 over the others, it is clearly the preferred choice because each realizes the other's predilection. This case is interesting because it leaves completely undetermined the question of with whom the predilection actually originated. We have here what is sometimes called a "bootstrap" mechanism: An effect arises, as it were, out of nothing but becomes reinforced through "feedback" into something definitive and stable.

One could object that the uniqueness of corner 6 is a strong factor to begin with. It is the only corner that is convex, as seen by the prisoner. Another example, mentioned by Anatol Rapoport in his foreword to Lefebvre's book, shows that the initial bias can be minimal and still lead to an almost certain outcome. Let two players guess the toss of a coin, and let them both win whenever their guesses coincide (regardless of the fall of the coin; in fact, no coin is needed in this game). Also let both players know that in a free choice between "heads" and "tails," a slightly larger number of people choose "heads." Whether this preponderance is small or large makes little difference in our game. Knowledge of even the slightest preference will make each player choose heads. In a sense each player anticipates the action of his "mirror image," since both face identical situations and since their interests coincide. Each concludes that his double will almost certainly choose "heads" because of its advantage, however small; therefore he will do the same.

The process is called *positive feedback*: If there is a tendency to go in a certain direction, the feedback will increase this tendency. Engineers are more concerned with *negative* feedback, which prevents a process from drifting away from an established norm. The classic example of negative feedback is the *governor* on a steam engine, a device which opens an escape valve when the pressure in the boiler becomes too high. The whole field of cybernetics began as a study of regulatory processes that use negative feedback.

If we were to replace the governor with a positive feedback device, the results might be disastrous. A pressure fluctuation above the norm would increase the setting on the burner, further raising the pressure. This would call for more heat and a more steeply rising pressure (Fig. 6.6) and lead to the eventual explosion of the boiler. Another example of positive feedback is a population of organisms whose rate of reproduction exceeds their death rate. In this case every increase in population size will cause an even steeper rise, resulting in a *population explosion*.

A more complex type of feedback is seen in the following example, taken again from Lefebvre's book. Two players, Petrov and Sidorov, are given choices, represented by the array shown in Fig. 6.7. Petrov must choose a (horizontal) row, Sidorov a (vertical) column in this array. The resulting wins or losses for each player are shown in the

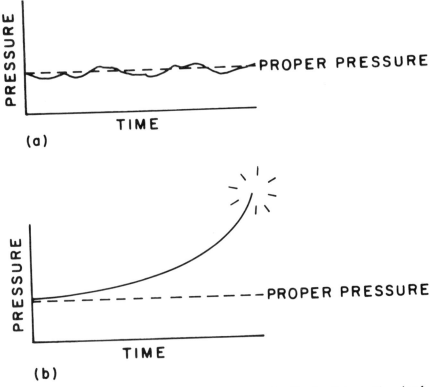

6.6 *Pressure control in a boiler. (a) Negative feedback; (b) positive feedback*

box where Petrov's row and Sidorov's column intersect. The first number in the box refers to Petrov, the second to Sidorov. Thus if Petrov chooses row A and Sidorov column D, the box labeled (−3, +5) indicates that Petrov loses three rubles, Sidorov wins five.

The choices reflect to some extent the temperament of the players. If Petrov is cautious, he may choose row A, in which he loses a little regardless of Sidorov's choice. If he is bold, he could take row B with the chance of winning five rubles (if Sidorov chooses column C), or losing ten (if Sidorov chooses column D). Sidorov runs similar risks. If both players are timid, they will lose two rubles each; but if they are both bold, they both lose ten. It is clearly of advantage to the bold player, who is intent on winning, to wear a "mask" of recklessness, thereby scaring his opponent into making the cautious choice. Let us say Petrov puts on a mask of fierce determination, but Sidorov is not fooled.

6.7 *Petrov versus Sidorov*

He happens to know that Petrov is really a timid person. This knowledge does not help Sidorov much, since he must assume that Petrov will go through with the bluff. (It would not be worth Petrov's efforts if in the end he, Petrov, made the timid choice. The whole masquerade could only reduce Petrov's losses from three rubles to two.)

For Sidorov to call Petrov's bluff and make the bold choice of column D is therefore likely to end in disaster for both. Sidorov's only chance in winning would lie in making sure Petrov *knows* that Sidorov knows that Petrov is putting on an act. Even then his choosing column D would be chancy.

What emerges from many but not all cases of reflexive dynamics is a special kind of indeterminacy which has to do with the fact that as we keep going around the loops, the light of logic dims rapidly and becomes less and less compelling. Where we stop in our chain of reasoning and where the opponent stops are thus fundamentally unpredictable. This indeterminacy is different from the one we encountered in the preceding section which was due to the chaotic microworld, or from the quantum indeterminacy we will treat in the next section.

The scenarios of these games seem somewhat contrived, but the complicated "reflexive dynamics," as well as the game advantage of projecting reckless determination, have all too real counterparts in the world in which we live. The following is an assessment of the nuclear balance of terror between the superpowers, taken from a *New York Times* editorial:

If we think *they* might launch a first strike on military targets, why shouldn't they think we might, particularly if we "stress" our capacity for selective strikes? And if both sides think that of the other, isn't one ultimately likely to try it before the other can?[6]

Note that these processes of assessing the motives and tendencies of others almost invariably involve self-reference—because *their* motives are contingent upon what *they* think *I* might do. That this is a general state of human affairs was expressed by Lefebvre:

In particular, a psychology that by-passes the problem of constructing the "inner worlds" of sentient beings or believes them to be deducible from observed physiological states appears inadequate. A sociology or a political science that ignores the effect of "knowing" the state of a system or the effect of publishing what one knows of that very state seems to neglect the most important distinction between the natural and the social sciences . . .[7]

The ubiquitous role of self-reference speaks to us from almost every work of art. Writers especially have been obsessed with the strange loops that are created when observer and observed become one. "To write," Ibsen once said, "is to sit in judgment of oneself." Julio Cortazar, in one of his delightful short stories, tells us of a man who becomes so intrigued with watching axolotls (salamanders), he winds up as an axolotl watching the man he was.

But art itself is recursive. Our demand that it be innovative propels art from movement to movement. Atonality in music, Dadaism in painting are examples of this strong bias toward self-avoidance in art. Sometimes the demand for innovation exceeds the inventiveness of the artists, and we are caught between gimmickry and banality.

We must ask ourselves finally about the nature of selfhood, not of a logical statement, or a mathematical equation, or art, but human selfhood from which all the others are derived. What is the nature of the *I* that contemplates itself, seeks itself, or avoids itself? Is it, perhaps, nothing but a product of its own self-contemplation, the work of a bootstrap process than can create something out of nothing?

This idea is attractive. It has been used in physics to account for the existence of elementary particles, and was invoked more recently to account for the origin of the universe itself. In what John Wheeler has called *self-reference cosmogony,* the universe is seen as originating in a singular event, the *big bang*, the *umbilicus* of everything that exists. But unlike other big-bang theories, Wheeler's universe is a *self-excited system*, brought into being by self-reference and contingent upon a physics that is just right for the eventual emergence of life and human consciousness. Past, present, and future are "wired together" in this universe in such a way that its birth is held up "until the blind accidents of evolution are guaranteed to produce, for some non-zero stretch of time in its history-to-be, the consciousness, and consciousness of consciousness, and communicating community, that will give *meaning* to that Universe from start to finish."[8]

The end Wheeler foresees is as dramatic as the beginning. He deems the eventual collapse of the universe inevitable, leading not to some continued though life-denying dynamics but simply the *end*. In Wheeler's words:

> Let a computing machine calculate onward instant by instant towards the critical moment, and let it make use of Einstein's standard 1915 geometrodynamics. Then a point comes where it cannot go on. Smoke, figuratively speaking, rises from the machine. Physics stops.

Not everyone agrees with Wheeler's self-reference cosmogony. Another contemporary physicist, Freeman Dyson, of Princeton University's prestigious Institute for Advanced Study, envisions a world that expands without limit and in which life can go on indefinitely.[9] The changing conditions in the expanding universe will demand, however, drastic changes in the scale and nature of life-forms. Conversely, the existence of intelligent life and, in particular, the existence of consciousness have a profound influence on the future evolution of Dyson's universe. Though fundamentally different, both Wheeler's and Dyson's cosmologies assign to consciousness decisive roles in the scheme of things.

Consciousness and physics

In the preceding sections I presented a picture of chaos and uncertainty. To these classical sources of confusion we must now add another: the indeterminacy, the fuzziness, the statistical character of the fundamental laws of physics as expressed by *quantum mechanics*. This revolutionary theory emerged around 1925 and is due mainly to the Danish physicist Niels Bohr, the Austrian Erwin Schrödinger, and the German Werner Heisenberg. If any understanding of the world or of ourselves is to emerge, it must be grounded firmly on the premises of quantum mechanics.

This theory represents the most radical and far-reaching departure from classical ideas since science began. It is not a capricious, far-out hypothesis but an inevitable change that was forced on physicists by incontrovertible facts. It is today a universally accepted scientific theory, although there is still some latitude in its interpretation and unresolved problems remain.

What is quantum mechanics? It grew out of the realization that waves such as light waves, X-rays, and others have under certain circumstances all the characteristics of particles: They are discrete units, localizable in space, and they carry fixed amounts of energy. At other times they have all the characteristics of waves. This duality was very puzzling at first. Then, in 1925 the French physicist De Broglie suggested that particles—for example, electrons—may also have the properties of waves. Soon, these *matter waves* were found in the laboratory. Also in 1925 Erwin Schrödinger proposed a new type of mechanics appropriate to these entities that combine wave and particle properties. It came to be known as *quantum mechanics.*

Among the concepts that soon emerged was a principle, named after Heisenberg, according to which objects could not be localized in space and time with arbitrary precision. This *uncertainty principle* tells us that particles move with an inherent fuzziness which allows us to specify only their probable locations, not where they "really" are.

Quantum mechanics has this probabilistic character throughout. But the real break with the past comes with the interpretation of these uncertainties, as proposed by the "Copenhagen school" and initiated primarily by Niels Bohr. The uncertainties, Bohr points out, are not merely an inadequate knowledge or understanding on our part; they concern nature itself. When the theory tells us that an electron has a 60 percent chance of being in one place and a 40 percent chance of being in another, our conventional notion would be that the electron "is really" at this moment in one place *or* the other, we just don't know which. The theory seems *incomplete*, since it only provides us with probabilities. Bohr, however, has shown it is no longer possible to speak of a reality that is independent of our knowledge. The particle is truly in a mixture of states, consisting of 60 percent of one location and 40 percent of the other. The theory is complete in its statement. Only when I look do I force the object into one *or* the other state. My observation has not just recorded reality, it has changed reality.

When does this strange interaction between observer and his object of study occur? According to Eugene Wigner, this happens "upon the entering of impressions into our consciousness."[10]

In classical mechanics, observations were carried out in a way that has been compared to looking at marine life through an underwater port of heavy plate glass, with the observer on one side, fish and shells on the other, unconcerned and undisturbed. We call the reality outside the glass port *objective*, because it appears to be unaffected by the observation and because it looks the same to any observer peering through that port.

The observer in the quantum-mechanical world is no longer able to peer unobtrusively through a plate of glass. He must reach out; he manipulates and *participates* in the goings-on he describes. In doing so he brings about unavoidable and generally unpredictable changes. It is this peculiar interaction between the consciousness of the observer, on the one hand, and physical reality, on the other, that dominates the stage in quantum mechanics.

The situation has been described by a bizarre example known as "Schrödinger's cat."[11] This hapless creature is locked in a box with a "hellish contraption" consisting of a small amount of radioactive substance, a Geiger counter, a hammer rigged to be released by the counter, and a glass vial of cyanide placed to be broken by the hammer. The sequence of events is thus: particle from decay of radioactive substance triggers Geiger counter, Geiger counter trips hammer, hammer smashes vial, cyanide escapes and kills cat.

However, all these events are hidden from view in the tightly closed box. Moreover, the time of occurrence cannot be predicted, since radioactive decay is an event for which quantum mechanics can only give probabilities. In the absence of an observation, the *complete* quantum-mechanical description of the radioactive substance would be that it has both decayed and *not* decayed, the counter both tripped and not tripped, the hammer both up and down, the vial both smashed and intact, the cat both dead and alive. Only when we take a look is the matter decided one way or the other, and it makes no sense to say that the situation was *really* that way *before* we looked.

All this flies in the face of common sense, which tells us that the cat can only be dead *or* alive but not both at once, and yet quantum mechanics leaves us little choice. The philosophical implications of this situation are still being debated, but one of the more exotic resolutions of the paradox is the so-called *many-world interpretation* of quantum mechanics. According to this view, the world literally *splits* into two or more different realities whenever a measurement is made. Each observation realizes each of the preexisting possibilities. But since these are now mutually exclusive, they coexist but in distinct, different worlds. The moment you open the box to check on Schrödinger's cat, there will be two different worlds, one in which you observe a healthy cat jumping out of the box, the other in which *another you* finds the cat poisoned.

The question of how our classical concepts of reality are affected by new developments in physics has recently come into sharper focus. In 1964 John S. Bell, a physicist at the European nuclear installation CERN in Geneva, published a paper pointing out that certain experimental tests might be used to decide whether or not quantum mechanics is really a complete description of nature as Bohr has proposed. If it is not, then a commonsense view of the world could somehow be restored. This was the belief firmly held by Albert Einstein. The critical tests involve something called Bell's inequality, a mathematical statement that must be satisfied if the commonsense view of the world is valid.

A number of experiments have now been performed, and the current evidence overwhelmingly indicates that Bell's inequality does not hold. We must accept the fact that nature is much stranger than we once thought. We must choose among alternatives that go against firmly held beliefs in science. One of these is the belief in an objective reality that is independent of a conscious observer, the other a principle called *locality*, according to which one physical event can cause another only if the second can be reached from the first by a signal traveling no faster than the speed of light.

The abandonment of the *principle of locality* was advocated by Bernard d'Espagnat of the University of Paris. He stated that "most particles or aggregates of particles that are ordinarily regarded as separate objects have interacted at some time in the past with other objects. The violation of separability seems to imply that in some sense all these objects constitute an indivisible whole. Perhaps in such a world the concept of an independently existing reality can retain some meaning, but it will be altered meaning and one remote from everyday experience."[12]

The strange *connectedness* which, according to d'Espagnat, exists between remote events, perhaps binding together all of the universe into an almost mystical unit, has been elaborated by others, especially in connection with the old problem of mind and consciousness and their relation to the material world. Speculations on this problem are of course tempting, but the issue remains murky. It is not unlikely, however, that physics may provide us with new surprises on this subject in the future.

To sum up this discussion on quantum mechanics, which the non-physicist must find strange and difficult to assimilate: The new laws of physics draw the observer onto the stage as an active participant in the spectacle his senses pick up. There is the strong suggestion that the dynamics of his consciousness may not be separable from the dynamics of the world.

We have labeled consciousness a *sensation*. It constitutes knowledge arrived at by introspection only. It is the most direct knowledge we have and the only knowledge which is indisputable. But what are the physical requirements? What biological or other equipment is necessary for the experience of consciousness? On that question we still have few clues. The guesses run all the way from *panpsychism*, according to which all objects in nature possess some measure of consciousness—perhaps in proportion to their complexity—to *solipsism*, which recognizes only one single being and one consciousness in the universe. Intermediate viewpoints attribute consciousness to all animals, to mammals only, to primates only, to humans only, and what was seriously suggested once—to men only.

If consciousness is a sensation it is also an *observation*, but of a rather special kind. Harold Morowitz, a biophysicist at Yale University, pointed out that here is a unique situation in which observer and system under observation are one and the same. He believed that under these conditions it is possible to perceive *microstates* of the system which would be inaccessible to an observer other than the self. He does not elaborate on the mechanisms for such observations or on the meaning that might be conveyed through them. I would modify this interesting idea somewhat. The states observed are not true microstates because the world of thermal noise carries no meaning. Instead they are the *ministates* which reflect the enormous number of subtle changes the nervous system has undergone in a lifetime of experience.

These states are *read* by dynamic processes akin to turbulence in the mechanics of fluids (see discussion on page 210), in which minute fluctuations are amplified and thus projected into the macroworld.

Another dynamic feature of consciousness is closely tied to the concept of self-reference. The frequently used term "self-consciousness" alludes to that. But self-reference, as we have seen, is also another source of uncertainty. Niels Bohr, in his famous essay entitled "Biology and Atomic Physics,"[13] speaks of "the impossibility in psychical experience to distinguish between the phenomena themselves and their conscious perception (which) clearly demands a renunciation of the simple causal description on the model of classical physics." Subject and object become indistinguishable because one mirrors the other in a self-referent cycle.

Thus it appears that every one of the uncertainties decreed by contemporary science plays a distinctive role in accounting for the phenomenon of consciousness. If this is so, then we may be able to answer in part the question raised above about the physical prerequisites of consciousness. If there is a necessary connection between consciousness and observation, and accepting that observation must be participatory according to quantum mechanics, then the most primitive requirement would be a system containing both sensors and effectors. If self-reference is necessary, then the system must have the ability to observe its own states. This would require loops in the processing of information. Finally, if we believe that chaotic dynamics is involved in fetching information from *ministates* to macrodynamics, then the system is required to have a complexity that allows for a large range of structural and dynamic scales.

7

LIKE A
SHEPHERD'S FIRE

Ulysses, wrapped up and sleeping under the leaves, like a shepherd's fire, is Ulysses nonetheless.

—*Alain* (ÉMILE AUGUSTE CHARTIER), The Gods

In this chapter I want to make some final comments on the man-machine analogy and the psychoneural identity theory, both of which have enjoyed considerable support in the scientific community. This chapter should not be taken as a summary of the preceding chapters. I meant the book to be a panorama of facts, views, and reflections, and I have made no pretense of presenting a unified or completed picture. What may appear to the reader now as isolated, and perhaps even conflicting propositions, will have to remain so, perhaps to be resolved at some future time.

James Clerk Maxwell, the nineteenth-century English physicist, had at one time been much preoccupied with the mind-body puzzle. Despairing of a solution, he somewhat testily referred to the problem as leading straight "through the den of the metaphysician, strewn with the bones of former explorers and abhorred by every man of science," and whose walls, I might add, are hung with the skins of many a scientist who should have known better. I will try to avoid a similar fate, not by being cleverer but by being more cautious and, like Clerk Maxwell, retreating in time.

* Perhaps there is no other route.—
which may also mean that all roads lead
to—and, simultaneously, from— Rome
Another loop?

The mess and the mystery

The idea that life, human life in particular, has the attributes of a machine stems undoubtedly from the human desire to understand. With understanding goes the power to manipulate, to control, and, ultimately, to create. Machines are human creations. To understand a system "as a machine" is to be able to create it. The machine concept of man, therefore, invests man with the powers of the Creator. At the same time, it lowers his stature to that of one of his own creations.

This dubious advantage has spurred man's efforts in two directions. His desire to assert his own supremacy by finding qualities no machine could duplicate is a constant challenge to his ingenuity to prove himself wrong.

About the middle of the eighteenth century, the idea took hold in France that one could dispense with Descartes's soul in the machine. This philosophy had many roots but was apparently prompted by a single discovery involving the lowly freshwater polyp, *Hydra*. In 1741 Abraham Trembley presented his startling findings to the French Academy of Sciences: *Hydra* was not a plant, as had been assumed up to that time, but an animal. But the most sensational part of Trembley's report concerned *Hydra*'s ability to regenerate: "For each portion of an animal cut in 2, 3, 4, 10, 20, 30, 40 parts, and, so to speak, chopped up, just as many complete animals are reborn, similar to the first."[1]

Trembley's discovery had a profound effect on French materialism. If the animal had a soul, it was argued, then cutting up *Hydra* must also cut up its soul. However, anything that could be sliced like this had to be *material*. These ideas became widely disseminated when in 1748 Julien Offray de la Mettrie published his famous *Man a Machine*. A century later the Austrian physicist Ludwig Boltzmann repeated a similar sentiment with the following Germanic sentence:

> Only when one admits that spirit and will are not something over and above the body, but rather complicated actions of material parts whose ability so to act becomes increasingly perfected by development, only when one admits that intuition, will and self-consciousness are merely the highest stages of development of these physico-chemical forces of matter by which primeval proto-

plasmic bubbles were enabled to seek regions that were more and avoid those that were less favorable for them, only then does everything become clear in psychology.[2]

Another century later, Monod stated it simply and categorically: "The cell is a machine, the animal is a machine. Man is a machine."

Just what is meant by "machine" is not always clear, but reference is usually made to whatever manmade contraption is the most sophisticated of its time. Today this honor must go to the electronic computer. The mathematician Norbert Wiener, who was very much involved in the computer revolution, defined a machine as "a device for converting incoming messages into outgoing messages."

A device can be specified by instructions or blueprints of some sort. The necessary information can be encoded in any number of ways, including a series of dots and dashes to be sent over a telegraph wire. The instructions must be of finite length, otherwise the device could never be built. Wiener elaborated on this idea by proposing that it is "conceptually" possible to specify all the design details that define a human being and literally send the man over a telegraph line.[3] (Children often think that sending flowers by wire involves this kind of dematerialization at one end and reassembly at the other.)

Of course, telegraph wires are obsolete now. The *teleporters* of modern science fiction have no conceptual difficulty with having an astronaut disappear in one place and reappear simultaneously on another planet. The purely technical problems seem almost trivial by today's standards.

Information is the specialty of our age. It saturates the air. It bounces back from our most distant planet. It is stored in enormous memory "banks" just in case some of it may be needed someday, when it can be retrieved with the push of a button and spewed out on a fast printer. Wiener's fantasy seems not at all remote. But is it realistic? We must ask again just *what* information would be required to duplicate a brain, and how this information could be acquired.

I have stressed repeatedly that a particular brain is distinguished from all others by three sets of criteria: genetic heritage, random and developmental influences, and the effects of *all* experiences which, beginning at birth, must have left their physical traces in the brain.

The first is the easiest to assess. Identical twins are identical in precisely this respect. Their DNA molecules, repositories of all genetic information, are identical. The codes contained in DNA can, in principle, be read by detailed chemical analysis or reproduced by chemical synthesis. The *cloning* of human beings, which is the reproduction of one or more genetically identical copies using only the information contained in the DNA of the original, is not yet a reality, but may be on the technological horizon.

The other two factors that make an individual are quite another matter. If it is true that random events affect details of brain circuitry, and that a least some of these changes become essential features of the functioning brain (see the discussion in Chapter 3 under the section called "Chance into essence"), then it becomes questionable whether means can ever be found to cull that information from a living brain and "materialize" it in another identical structure. Finally, the enormous amount of information contained in the network of associations, conditioning, and recoverable memories each of us carries in his head appears to be equally inaccessible. I believe these intrinsic difficulties in "reading out" the appropriate information are more severe than the problem of "handling" the information once it is acquired, although that is not to be belittled either. The information may be so massive as to require thousands of years to be transmitted over a modern high-speed computer line.

The case of the "split-brain" patient, Paul, described by Gazzaniga (pages 190–191) shows how extremely subtle differences affect personality. The patient was unusual in that both brain hemispheres possessed a considerable language faculty. When asked their job preferences, the left side answered "draftsman," the right "car racing." The two brain halves are, of course, genetically identical. They have also, until the time of their surgical separation, shared all sensory experiences and have partaken in all actions of the individual. Why, then, the different behavior? And why did the surgeon's knife going through the *corpus callosum* produce two separate, nonidentical conscious beings? It is Trembley's problem again, raised to a much higher level.

Is it necessary that living beings be constructed of biological molecules, and composed of cells, blood vessels, and nerves? Must brains be made of neurons, or would a *functionally equivalent* system do as well?

Freeman Dyson, who speculated on some exotic life-forms in an eternally expanding universe, asks whether the basis of consciousness is *matter* or *structure*. "If I could make a copy of my brain with the same structure, but using different materials, would the copy think it was me?"[4] Of course, we don't know whether the copy would think at all, since we don't know enough about the relationship between structure and thought. But if it did think, my guess is that it would not identify with *me*. After all, identical twins have separate personalities, and even split brains, though identical in genetic makeup *and* experience, have independent consciousnesses. A little thought experiment may further convince us of the impossibility of merging selfhoods. If my perfect copy identifies with me, then it follows that I should identify with *it*. If one has to be destroyed, it should make no difference to me which one of us is to survive. But it does.

We must be careful when we replace things with what we believe are their equivalents. Lefebvre tells us of a "game" in which two adversaries face each other with pistols. Each is promised one ruble if he shoots the other. It is presumed that no moral or legal stigma is attached to killing. A player may go through the following reasoning: "Whether I shoot him or not will not affect his decision to shoot. I may as well shoot, then, to get the ruble in case he doesn't shoot." But then he realizes that his opponent, facing the same dilemma, must have come to the same conclusion. Both will die in the hope of getting one ruble. This is silly; hence he will change his mind and decide not to shoot, knowing that his opponent will reason likewise. But if his opponent will not shoot, he figures, he might as well shoot and win the ruble. And so on.

The two are so alike that Lefebvre feels justified in replacing one with the mirror image of the other. Here is what happens:

> X lifts his pistol and sees that the image of his "opponent" does the same and that the expression on his face is menacing. X understands that if he presses the trigger, the image will, too. X lowers the pistol. The "opponent" does the same.
>
> "I shall now fool him," thinks X, "since he, too, must see the same sort of image." Immediately a sly expression appears on the face of the image and a preparatory movement of the pistol . . .[5]

To come back to Dyson's question, there is still the same fundamental barrier to our knowing the details of our brain structure before we can provide that structure with a new material representation. This barrier may be unsurmountable.

Another conjecture has it that life and consciousness somehow emerge at a certain level of complexity of information processing. According to this belief, some future computer will cross the line that separates the obedient machine from living, thinking beings, and we may have the evolution of a new life-form,-the *living computer*.

Such an idea certainly cannot be ruled out. There is no reason (that we know of) why life could not be sustained by material forms radically different from those involving biomolecules and cells. But we must caution against the naïve belief that we are now justified in expecting human cognitive functions in a machine of our design. Descartes's *cogito ergo sum* should not be perverted into "it is, therefore it thinks."

One thing we all deplore about our lives is their finiteness. Why must our bodies weaken with age and die? We look with envy at our electronic marvels with their exchangeable plug-in modules which give them a virtually limitless lifetime. A comparison between the two systems points up some further differences. The physical part of the computer—its *hardware*, as it is called—is a closed system. Its elements, the integrated-circuit "chips," have precisely specified functions which they must perform unerringly until they fail. They are then replaced by fresh units with the same functions. The only modifiable parts of the computer are the *programs*, the "software," which tell the computer what to do.

In the living brain we know of no such distinction. The brain does not follow instructions, it simply *functions*. Nietzsche remarked that "a thought comes when 'it' wills, not when I will." Memory, motivation, associations—all the changes which in a computer would require instructions occur in the brain as a result of changes in the structure itself—the hardware. In this sense the brain is an *open system*. Not only is material continuously flowing in and out of every cell, but the structure itself undergoes continuous modification as it interacts with the world around it and with itself. And since information now resides in the structure itself, a fresh plug-in module just won't do.

This is not to say that structural changes do not occur in machines. They may even be used to advantage. In the running-in phase of an automobile, its moving parts fit themselves into the mechanism by wear, thus improving the performance. Self-structuring is used in some advanced electronic designs, but no machine of our making has its essential features so embodied in a self-made and reflexive structure. Unlike any machine existing or contemplated, brains cannot be replaced, duplicated, or even reset. Thus not only is every brain unique, so is every moment in a brain's life.

Henrik Ibsen's tragic character, Peer Gynt, at the end of his life is concerned about the preservation of his selfhood. He pleads with the Devil to take him, seeing this as his only chance for immortality. He is told, instead, to resign himself to the "casting ladle," that is, oblivion. The Devil asks:

> . . . What good
> Would it be to you if I offered you board and
>   lodging?
> Think a minute. You're a sensible man.
> You'd keep your memory, that's true enough,
> But what have you got to remember?
> I promise you, the memory of things past
> Would give you little joy.
> You'd find no cause for weeping or for laughter,
> No cause for rejoicing or despair,
> They'd merely be a source of irritation.[6]

Selfhood cannot be perpetuated forever. If the system becomes closed, it would indeed seem a source of irritation to have to gnaw on the same store of memories forever. If it remains open, adding new experiences to the old, the memory banks of the brain must sooner or later become filled, and old memories will have to be cast off. There will come a time when all connections with the former self will have ceased.

Perhaps the outstanding behavioral quality of man is what has been called his capacity for "self-transcendence." Born with all the drives and desires for "creature comfort" he shares with animals, he is likely to forsake these in pursuit of what he conceives to be his self-image, whether heroic, adventurous, messianic, or just plain different. The human self is to a large extent self-assembled. This was expressed beautifully 500 years ago by Pico della Mirandola, a Renaissance scholar who delivered in 1486 in Rome his celebrated "Oration on the Dignity of Man." At the end of Creation, Pico tells us, all specific roles had been assigned, all ecological niches filled, to use modern jargon. But "the Divine Artificer still longed for some creature which might comprehend the meaning of so vast an achievement, which might be moved with love at its beauty and smitten with awe at its grandeur." He solves the dilemma by giving man "nothing wholly his own" except the capacity to make himself into anything he, man, fancies. Pico describes the final act of Creation:

Taking man, therefore, this creature of indeterminate image, He set him in the middle of the world and thus spoke to him: "We have given you, oh Adam, no visage proper to yourself, nor any endowment properly your own, in order that whatever place, whatever form, whatever gifts you may, with premeditation, select, these same you may have and possess through your own judgement and decision. The nature of all other creatures is defined and restricted within laws which We have laid down; you, by contrast, impeded by no such restrictions, may, by your own free will, to whose custody We have assigned you, trace for yourself the lineament of your own nature. I have placed you at the very center of the world, so that from that vantage point you may with greater ease glance round about you on all that the world contains . . .[7]

The following story provides an intriguing contrast to Pico della Mirandola's portrait of man. It is taken from a television drama that appeared some years ago in a series called *The Twilight Zone*. The story begins as a small-time gambler is shot to death in a street fight. A limousine pulls up. An urbane elderly gentleman emerges, motions at the prostrate figure of the dead gambler. He rises, is taken into the limousine and driven to a plush casino-hotel.

There he finds everything he ever wanted but never achieved in his life. Comfort, elegance, beautiful, accommodating women, and unvarying luck at the gambling tables.

The urbane gentleman asks whether he finds everything to his liking. No complaints at first. But after a few blissful days he finds it all too much. Gambling is no fun, the gambler complains, if you know you're always going to win. His host is eager to oblige. "We can let you lose now and then," he suggests. "Say every third or fourth time? Tell me *exactly* what you like, and I will arrange it for you."

"No, no, you don't understand," said the exasperated gambler. "Besides, it is all a mistake. I shouldn't even be here. I should be in the other place."

"And what makes you think this is not the other place?" asks the urbane gentleman.

The gambler's difficulty in defining life is analogous to the efforts of the practitioners of artificial intelligence to catalogue the functions of the human brain. The elusiveness of both may just be our familiarity with them. Or, as Einstein remarked, "What does a fish know about the water in which he swims all his life?" On the other hand, the inability to be defined or prescribed may be part of the very essence of life, at least of intelligent life.

Between dualism and identity theory

Mind is a troublesome word. We have inherited it from the Latin *mens*. However, we look in vain for its equivalent in some other languages. In German we have *Seele* (soul), *Geist* (spirit), *Verstand* (intellect), *Vernunft* (reason), *Gemüt* (disposition), *Gedächtnis* (memory), *Meinung* (opinion), *Absicht* (intent)—but no word has all the shades of meaning of *mind*. In general, we have no difficulty in the use of the word. The context makes clear which of the above or other meanings are intended. But trouble arises when we try to *define* mind or make pronouncements about its relationship with the brain.

It would be foolish to conclude that the mind-body problem is just a linguistic-semantic difficulty. The concept of "mind" is useful when we want to refer collectively to a great variety of states that we either observe by introspection or surmise in others by observing their behavior.

The various aspects of mind appear to form some sort of hierarchy with *sensations* the most elementary ingredients. To have a sensation (of sight or sound or touch) seems neither reducible to other phenomena nor open to question. And yet the nature of this most direct channel we have to the outside world was recently questioned by Donald O. Hebb, one of today's outstanding psychologists.[8] Hebb doubts that there exists "an immediate, introspective acquaintance with our own mental processes." He states that "it cannot even be safely assumed that visual sensation is recognizably distinct from auditory or tactile sensation, intrinsically and apart from the context in which it occurs." He cites as an example the case of "facial vision," a sensation of spatial awareness people report having in total darkness and often interpret as a form of vision. It is now attributed to the auditory phenomenon of *echolocation*. Hebb concludes that "we do not perceive our sensations or perceptions but instead the thing sensed or perceived." The argument is reminiscent of Gibson's theory of affordances (pages 160–163). But the example is not very representative. The subtle sounds in the dark room and their modification by the presence of nearby objects are barely at the perceptual level. The subject is more aware of his conclusions ("the thing sensed") than of the sensations. Counterexamples come to mind easily. Sometimes with unusual or incomplete combinations of sensations, the "thing sensed" may elude the observer. He may be aware of his sensations and his own puzzlement —the "What was that?" reaction. Under more typical conditions the source is correctly identified, as are the sensations that inform us about it. During a thunderstorm we have no difficulty telling the thunder from the lightning, even if the *thing sensed* is one and the same.

Hebb's statement is at odds also with observations on split-brain patients, where, as we have seen (pages 190–191), there can be a transmission of moods between cerebral hemispheres without communication of the underlying causes. In the case of sensations coming from our own bodies, the perception more often than not is of the sensations, not their causes.

To say that sensations are not perceived is almost self-contradictory. Unfortunately, the word *sensation* lacks an appropriate verb. The verb *to sense* directs attention to the sensory apparatus and its physical response rather than to the subjective experience of a sensation. We would not even consider it a metaphor to say that a smoke detector *senses* the presence of a fire. But nobody would say it is "having a sensation." Perhaps the word *feel* conveys better the essentially subjective quality we need here, but its usage becomes awkward in describing anything other than skin or body sensations.

We have touched here on one facet of the mind-body problem. To sense as a smoke detector senses is an understandable, transparent function of matter. To "have a sensation" (of pleasure or pain) brings in consciousness, moods, and thoughts. We say it involves the mind. But it also involves neural messages and firing patterns, distributions of brain hormones, enzymes, and transmitter substances.

We can *talk* about two types of phenomena taking place in the cranium. But are these really two? Or is one or the other fictitious? Or are they one and the same? To make a very sweeping classification of views, a positive answer to the first question would characterize the *dualist* position. "Yes" to the second question marks one of the *monist* viewpoints. "Yes" to the last question is the position taken by the *psychoneural identity theory*.

Dualism has had many proponents in the course of time, but the best-known formulation is undoubtedly that of René Descartes. In his view the body, which includes the brain, is adequately described by a machine. All processes taking place there are subject to rigidly deterministic physical laws. Mind and all things mental constitute a world apart from the physical system and obey dynamic laws of their own. The two realms are thus quite disinct except that they interact at one point, which Descartes believed to be the pineal body, a small cone-shaped gland at the base of the brain. Here the mind can make things happen in the physical brain through the act of volition, and the brain in turn can "convey" things to the mind.

This form of dualism has two weaknesses: It precludes for all mental processes the kind of understanding we have been demanding in scientific "explanations" of physical phenomena, and it allows the non-physical phenomena of mind to have at least *some* effect on the dynamics of the physical brain. Whether or not one finds this *metaphysical* intrusion into physical laws disturbing is a matter of temperament. It would certainly be unacceptable to anyone believing in *scientific reductionism*, the doctrine according to which *all* phenomena are ultimately reducible to generally valid physical laws. On the other hand, some scientists, especially those having a strong religious conviction, may find dualism a quite palatable philosophy.

Monisms, by contrast, recognize only one of the two realms. Materialist monisms tend to reject the legitimacy of questions regarding such introspective qualities as consciousness and sensations, and concentrate instead on the observable behavior of the individual and his brain. Eddington had an expression for it: "What my net won't catch isn't fish."

Idealist monisms often deny the reality of the physical world and make the human "spirit" and its various manifestations the only unquestioned elements of existence. Here a different net catches different fish.

We finally come to the psychoneural identity theory, which is the current rage among philosophers and neuroscientists. It is a merger of monism and dualism: There is the physical brain, and it obeys physical laws; there are mental phenomena, including all the introspectively accessible shades of mood and thought. But the two realms are really one. All mental qualities are contained in the material disposition of the central nervous system. The theory is, therefore, also called *central state materialism*. My perception of a visual scene *is* a spatiotemporal sequence of events in my brain. The memory of having observed a similar scene *is* another "brain state." My joy at seeing you *is* yet another brain state.

Herbert Feigl, one of the outstanding proponents of the psychoneural identity theory, speaks of two kinds of knowledge: that derived from one's own introspective acquaintance with one's brain states—he calls it *"knowledge by acquaintance"*—and *"knowledge by description,"* that which is derived through communication of some sort.[9] The names *sentience* and *sapience* have also been applied to these two states.

Let us now take a closer look at the states to be compared. We have the physical states, known to us by description, and the mental states, known by acquaintance. For either state there exist broad categories within which we have almost limitless variety and detail. It is not difficult to convince oneself that a *correlation* exists between broad categories of brain states and equally broadly defined mental states. Recent studies on blood flow and glucose consumption in the brain, when it is engaged in different tasks (page 75), give more than a hint in that direction. Here specific regions in the neocortex "light up" under different physical and mental tasks.

When we speak of a *correlation*, we mean that a given (broadly defined) mental state is usually accompanied by a certain (equally broadly defined) neuronal state. But what about the *details* of neuronal activity and the *whole* content of the mental state? We know next to nothing about the first. In the case of the second, the difficulty of any attempt to describe or even to scrutinize the contents of the mind becomes itself a new mental state and hence alters irreversibly the very thing one is trying to grasp. Back to quantum mechanics.

We become aware of the fact that the terms "mental state" and "physical state" are very poor terms for phenomena involving continuously changing forms. It is better to speak of two dynamic processes which we must compare and which the psychoneural identity theory tells us are identical.

For the mental processes a detailed dynamic description is not even conceivable. The intrinsic difficulties in obtaining detailed neuronal dynamics, or even the complete instantaneous "frozen" state of the nervous system, have been discussed. They stem from the impossibility of measuring microstates of a macroscopic system. We have also pointed out that detailed neural dynamics are not likely to evolve in a calculable way.

We now have two dynamic processes, but no means of ascertaining detailed descriptions of either. What is worse, we do not know whether the instantaneous state of one should be compared with a simultaneous state in the other or with one preceding or following the first. The experiments by Benjamin Libet (page 197) suggest that the consciousness of a neural event (stimulation of skin receptors) does not occur until certain other processes have taken place in the central nervous system, and it is then *referred back* to the time of the sensory event. While this argument does not preclude an identity between simultaneous mental and physical states, it raises very delicate questions regarding the real time of occurrence of a mental event.

The psychoneural identity theory is a radical extension of the *psychoneural linking hypothesis.* According to this much weaker assumption, neural and mental processes can be linked or *paired.* We are not asking whether they are identical or which is the cause of the other. Psychophysical linking seems at first glance to be the inevitable precondition for any rational scientific approach to the subject of mental processes. Unfortunately, even this weak assumption cannot be accepted without some reservations. As before, we have no means of describing the processes to be linked except in very broad terms. Even at that level, differences are found in the meaning of brain states from one individual to another. We may account for this variability by noting that there are differences in neural circuitry from person to person. Some of these differences may be genetic, some developmental, and others may reflect the individual's particular set of experiences going all the way back to infancy. The individual differences in the "linkage" between mental and brain states are expected to become more profound as we increase the detail in the description of the states. Sooner or later we would arrive at a point where the linkage is not even reproducible for the same person, because the intervening experience would have produced changes in the physical system that may affect the "mapping" between the physical and the "mental."

Ultimately neither a physical nor a mental state will ever be repeated in all details. We can state this categorically, since the physical system of the brain is changing with every addition to its memory store, and since the sensory inputs will never be precisely the same at any two moments in a person's life. In the strictest sense then, the psychoneural linking hypothesis tells us only that a particular mental state and a particular neuronal state (neither precisely ascertainable) have coexisted in one individual at one instant. Additional meaning can be recovered only as we broaden (make fuzzier) our definitions of neural and mental states.

What I said above about the linking hypothesis applies equally to the identity theory. But the identity theory, at least in its currently promulgated versions, suffers from another inherited flaw. Descartes originated the idea of a body that was nothing but a machine, operating on the then-known simple physical laws. In addition, he postulated that a "soul" inhabited that body. Modern identity theory removes the soul, but substitutes nothing more sophisticated for Descartes's seventeenth-century concept of the body-machine. It is still a machine, and classical mechanics of a rather pedestrian variety is pressed into service to provide a model for mental phenomena. It is not surprising that the results of this "promissory materialism," as the philosopher Karl Popper has called it, provide little intellectual comfort. Leibnitz's comment on the theme is still valid: "A man goes out of his house, looks in at the window, and is surprised to find that the room is empty."

The primitive state of contemporary materialism is only slightly exaggerated by Owen St. John, who chides Monod for "describing the world of experience as bits of matter moved by mechanical law and nothing more".[10] At another point he says, "A dead and mechanical world of matter, as conceived by Cartesian physics, cannot conceivably produce life by doing the only thing it has the power to do, namely, redistributing itself in space."

We can gain a perspective on Cartesian physics by reminding ourselves that Sir Isaac Newton was a boy of eight when Descartes died. It sometimes appears that what has happened since that time in the field of physics is equally unappreciated by the materialist philosopher, who leans on it, and his critic, who damns it. The richness of phenomena in the physics of today and the depths of the problems that still remain go far beyond anything anticipated only a few decades ago. A few of these topics were taken up in Chapter 6. I mentioned how the chaos of the microcosm can impinge on macrodynamics, and how events on a cosmic scale may affect events in everyday life. I referred briefly to quantum mechanics and the novel relationship it established between a system under observation and its observer. I mentioned recent experiments showing a violation of Bell's inequality and some of the bizarre conclusions physicists have drawn from that. Of causality and determinism, once the foundations of natural science, J. M. Jauch, another contemporary physicist, says that they are "in fact a gigantic prejudice which is often wrongly identified with the very essence of science."

Among the nonmaterial phenomena occupying physicists today there are the still unresolved properties of time and space, including the rich phenomenology of empty space—the vacuum state.[11] Finally, there are conjectures that the origin or the evolution of the universe at large may be dependent on its compatibility with intelligent life. It is a paradox that at a time when physicists find themselves unable to discuss the dynamics of the universe without involving human consciousness as a direct participant, materialist philosophers can still claim that mind is *nothing but* the *"mechanical sprouting"* of a machine.

But dualism seems equally obsolete. Descartes can be pardoned for invoking the soul, since the physics of his day couldn't do much more than turn a waterwheel. But as we near the end of the twentieth century, physics has provided us with an embarrassment of conceptual riches that makes any metaphysical assumption seem superfluous.

Are we able, then, to "explain" mental phenomena with our enriched collection of physical laws? This would be the hope of an enlightened reductionist. But it is much too early to be sure that such a *science of the mind* will eventually emerge. The laws are still too confused and the mysteries too deep. It is possible also that the phenomenon of sensation, which I have taken as central to any discussion of mind, will turn out to be not *derivable* from any physical laws but embedded in the foundation of a future formulation of natural science.

8

EPILOGUE: GARAPOCAIA

We have art in order not to die of the truth.

—F. NIETZSCHE

A very personal story

In the beginning of this book I raised the question what it is to be human. In searching for an answer we examined the brain, that superb instrument of reason. I also made a plea for a rational or scientific approach to the world around us and the problems confronting us. I expressed my dismay at the amount of irrationality and superstition that are again sweeping our society.

But if reason is a human attribute, it does not follow that irrationality is inhuman. On the contrary, a predilection toward the occult has dominated human affairs throughout history more than science has. The most rational human gets carried away by a good mystery yarn. Whether we admit it or not, there is a bit of shaman in each of us. It is therefore not inappropriate to insert here a chapter of personal history that brings out this odd human duality. The events I will relate happened almost forty years ago, but they have had a powerful bearing on my intellectual development.

The people involved would probably, if they were still alive, disagree with most of the ideas I have expressed, and I was likewise—during my short stay in Garapocaia—locked with them in an intense struggle of ideas. And yet, between exasperation and desperation, I have always felt profound compassion and love for the strange group of people whose lives briefly crossed mine in the early days of World War II on an incredibly beautiful island off the coast of Brazil.

I had just turned twenty, lived alone in Rio de Janeiro, was out of money and out of a job. My circumstances were such that I could not afford to hesitate when friends informed me of an opening as farm laborer (the job initially involved mostly cleaning stables) on an island off the coast to the south. A short formal letter, in which I applied for the job, was answered promptly by a certain Reimar von Bülow-Radum, a Danish millionaire, who owned the plantation by the name of "Garapocaia." I should not decide hastily, the letter stated. It was a big step. Life on the island was hard, not just because of the hard labor that would be expected of me. Not even the great natural beauty would be able to soften the impact of what he called "the awful confrontation with one's self." The letter went on to introduce the other people there: his wife Mina, Italian (she was a countess Taon di Revel, but he did not tell me that in his letter); Leonya, a Russian émigré, who was the administrator of the plantation; and an unhappy young lad of German parentage by the name of Kurt Kriechle, who performed the duties I would be taking over and who was about to be sacked.

My pay would be ten *milreis* a month, which in Rio would not have supported me for more than a day, plus room and board. The low pay was to make sure that nobody would take the job just for the money. If I were still interested I should write, sending my date of birth including the hour, if I knew it. The oddity of the letter did not fully strike me at the time. I was too elated at the prospect of a steady income, however paltry.

A few days later a rusty old coastal steamer with the unlikely name of *Aspirante Nascimento* took me south. We stopped at a number of small ports on the way: Angra dos Reis, Ubatuba, Caraguatatuba. I remember Angra in particular because it had a haunting, timeless quality about it, with its low colonial buildings clustered tightly around the small port and the green wall of the jungle behind it. When I returned to Brazil more than thirty years later, I was told that it is now the site of a large nuclear power station. I refrained from revisiting it.

We arrived in São Sebastião well past midnight. I was met there by three Indians who took me across the strait to the island in a large dugout canoe. An envelope handed to me contained a short greeting, some money to pay the men, and instructions to tell them to beat the oars against the canoe on arrival at Garapocaia. It was signed "Reimar."

It was almost three A.M.—they had been rowing steadily. Suddenly they stopped, and one of the rowers began to pound the side of the canoe rythmically with his oar. In days to come I was to use this form of communication myself many times. The hollow, resonant thuds can be heard for miles. At first, I could discern no sign of land in the utter blackness before us. Then a light appeared and slowly approached. A man carrying a Coleman lantern was walking on what was evidently a strip of beach just ahead of us. A dog barked and soon became visible too in the light of the lantern.

A short gravel walk between giant selloums and a row of pandanus trees took us to a sprawling old house. Once inside, Senhor Reimar began, without further introduction, to read to me from a stack of typewritten sheets that were arranged before him on a huge table. It was some kind of character sketch of a young man with whom I did not identify at first. I remember being hungry and waiting for him to ask me whether I wanted something to eat.

I must have nearly dozed off a few times during the lengthy reading, but suddenly I came awake with a start. The man who had hired me to clean his stables was reading me my horoscope. I was convinced that he was quite mad, and that I had spent the last of my savings to deliver myself into the hands of a lunatic.

During the next few months, the feeling of alarm I had experienced that first night slowly gave way to panic and later to quiet despair. My duties in the stables, oppressive as they were, were only a small aspect of my mission in Garapocaia. I was to be a link in a chain of events controlled by a man known as the *Tibetan*. The Tibetan occupied a position near the top of a hierarchical structure that directed the destinies of humans all over the globe. Reimar modestly described his own position in the pyramid as very minor.

The identity and whereabouts of the Tibetan were not known at the level of our small spiritual enclave in Garapocaia, but instructions would filter down continually through a network of intermediaries, confirmed by occasional letters from a composer in Finland and a woman novelist in London. Apart from these few tangible communications, the network operated entirely by *thought transmission*, according to Reimar. To my frequent queries regarding the nature of the transmissions, he would only say that it was not necessary to write. "We just *know*."

I should mention that, apart from a good Central European secondary education, my background at that time included no professional training in the sciences. The skepticism with which I reacted to all this was therefore a personally felt *disbelief* rather than a defense of any well-formulated natural philosophy of my own. This disbelief threatened my personal integrity, inasmuch as everyone around me —Reimar, Mina, Leonya, and even young Kurt Kriechle—accepted with unquestioning faith their assigned roles in this spiritual network.

My condition would have been tolerable though unpleasant if I could have dismissed the goings-on lightly. What really aggravated my plight was the profound admiration I began to develop for the three main characters. Reimar, besides being rich and aristocratic (and having a noble contempt for both attributes), was a concert pianist who at the height of a successful career as an artist in Europe decided he despised playing before audiences, took his nine-foot Bechstein to Garapocaia, and retired. Mina, far from her ducal palace in Torino, was tending our vegetable gardens, her health undermined by a host of tropical diseases. Leonya, a gentle bear of a man, was the plantation's factotum. His competence was boundless. He knew how to forge horseshoes, treat cattle against scores of parasites and other diseases, wage a continual battle against the leaf-cutting sauva ants, build roads, and navigate the often-treacherous straits to the mainland. Every piece of machinery purred obediently under his hand. He not only spoke, he *mastered* the six languages spoken in Garapocaia, in addition to his own native Russian.

The library at Garapocaia was an important facility, and I was urged to make full use of it. The selections were, of course, somewhat one-sided. I remember struggling through Count Hermann Keyserling's ponderous and occultist *Reisetagebücher*, an English novel entitled *Om*, whose author I have forgotten, and a strange story called *Winged Pharaoh*, by Joan Grant, allegedly written by a young woman who recalled her life as a pharaoh some millennia ago. Then there were several shelves of Russian émigré literature, some of it in English translation. They were rather hackneyed escapist tales (no Nabokov among them) in which the Bolshevik revolution in the end always faded away like a bad dream. Halfway through the stories it usually turned out that the Czar was not really dead but hiding out somewhere, waiting for a glorious return.

I remember one scene describing a religious service being held secretly somewhere at the height of the revolution. The priest told the congregation that Russia could be saved, but only if *one* member could be found whose conscience was free of guilt. Several of the parishioners came forward, but when they were told by the priest to touch a cross, their hands turned red with blood. A small child was ushered forward. Surely he would save them. But, no, he had betrayed his father to the Soviets, and his hands, too, turned scarlet at the touch of the cross. Just when everybody despaired, a tall blond youth slowly approached the altar, touched the cross, then turned to the congregation and raised his white palms. Russia was saved.

Another novel that left a strong impression on me was entitled *Behind the Thistles*. It depicted the revolution advancing to ever higher levels of violence and inhumanity, and the eventual complete breakdown of the society. The country is finally swept by waves of deadly epidemics. Europe, in fear of a spreading plague, closed all borders with Russia. Soon the no-man's-land is overgrown with a thick growth of thistles. *Behind the Thistles*, all life is presumed to have ceased. This state of affairs lasts for some years. Occasional attempts by small parties to penetrate the thistle barrier always end in failure. It is again a tall blond youth, who had fled to Paris as a child, who one day receives a telepathic message that he must brave the thistle fields and return to Russia. He does and finds not a dead wasteland but an incredibly advanced society led by a benevolent Czar, ready now to reveal itself to the rest of the world.

I did not know it at first, but I was being groomed to fill Leonya's position as Garapocaia's administrator, since personal circumstances made it necessary for him to contemplate leaving the island in the near future. Under his tutelage I forged horseshoes, milked the cows, mixed their feed, and inspected them for ticks and festering insect bites. Meanwhile, Reimar, concerned with my spiritual development, set about the task of my conversion, gently but systematically, starting from the moment of my arrival and the reading of my horoscope. His patience in this endeavor was most disconcerting to me, since it hinted at a large reservoir of strength.

The strength of my own position was not helped by the physical circumstances in which I found myself. We always met in the evening when Reimar came out of the music room and I returned from the stable. He had a way, which I found particularly annoying, of casually mentioning some outrageously impossible event and then waiting for my reaction. Then I, painfully aware of the aura of cow dung that hung about me, would argue that there had to be a perfectly sound explanation for the phenomenon. (To this day I have always excluded the possibility of even the slightest intellectual dishonesty on Reimar's part.)

Here is a small sample of the continual stream of strange tales to which I was subjected. On the subject of horoscopes, Reimar claimed to have had convincing proof of their validity. He had worked extensively on his own horoscope, but had been frustrated. "At first, I did not recognize myself," he told me. But then he discovered that a shift of only two hours in his supposed time of birth produced exactly the person he judged himself to be. His mother had maintained that the first time was the correct one. Years later, he discovered letters she had written at the time he was born. The hour mentioned coincided with that of *his* horoscope.

In his youth Reimar had lived in London and, besides pursuing his musical career, dabbled in painting. He found an insignificant-looking canvas at a dealer and immediately *knew* he had to buy it. After cautiously and expertly removing a layer of paint, he uncovered—a Constable! It was there now in the living room in Garapocaia, massive, mysterious, beautiful.

One night, late, Reimar, Leonya, and I were sitting in that room. The night was particularly oppressive and even the usually lively sounds from the jungle outside seemed stifled by the heat. Leonya and Reimar were exchanging glances whose significance escaped me. Finally, Reimar nodded to Leonya and said, "You feel it too, don't you?" He looked impressive sitting there in the light of a kerosene lamp, gaunt, with the Constable as a backdrop. "Feel what?" asked the stableboy. Leonya answered for him: "Lampert."

Now, Lampert was a furtive little man, probably a haunted man, whom I had met on a few occasions in the village. He was Austrian and had held the position of administrator at Garapocaia before Leonya. He had taken readily to Reimar's occult teachings and, according to Reimar, had become quite adept at some of the practices. But his motives were evil, I was told, and he had become dangerous. When he was dismissed, he left the plantation but not the island. All this had happened before my arrival there, but the name *Lampert* was always mentioned with the certain delicacy some people reserve for the name of the Devil.

I had met Lampert a few times in my travels around the island. He was always anxious to hear the latest news from Garapocaia and frequently expressed his bitterness at not being in charge there anymore. "With these," he told me repeatedly, raising a pair of incongruously large hands, "I have built Garapocaia." He recalled with great nostalgia the years when he and Reimar carved the plantation out of malaria-infested jungle, and he bitterly resented Leonya as a Johnny-come-lately on the island.

On this occasion Leonya explained that Lampert was evidently, and with evil intent, making his presence felt. I reacted with more than my usual amount of cynicism. I, too, felt depressed from the heat. But this was too much. Reimar only smiled. A week later he came through the stable. I was sitting on a stool milking a cow named Mascote. "I saw Lampert in the village today," Reimar told me. Then he waited for me to ask what Lampert had to say. I did, but I already knew the answer —a strong argument for precognition if you are so inclined. I could have predicted every single word. "He told me he was thinking of us last week. Wanted to know whether we felt it," Reimar answered and walked away.

In retrospect, the most puzzling aspect about my stay at Garapocaia was that I did not sooner or later succumb to the lure of the occult instead of engaging as I did in an unhappy and wholly one-sided struggle against it. Only once and very briefly did I waver, and I felt rather sorry for Reimar because he thought my conversion had come.

The occasion was a brief but violent bout with malaria. I was put up in a small guest room next to Reimar's music room. A candle was burning next to my bed, and Reimar sat there talking to me most of the night. I was delirious, and I don't remember much of what he said, but I have a clear recollection of a dream I had toward morning. I was back in Europe, which I had left not so long ago and for which I had lately developed an intense longing, together with an equally intense dislike of my present circumstances on the island. But in my dream it was a hostile and frightening Europe, and I remember a feeling of terrible loss and sadness at having left Garapocaia. When I awoke the sun was already up, the air was crisp through the open window, and my fever was broken. I felt very much at peace and didn't want to be anywhere else. But as I was telling Reimar about the dream, I knew that its significance would appear larger to him than it did to me, and I almost regretted feeling so clear-headed about it.

The peace, too, turned out to be short-lived. Soon the battle of wits started again. It took some strange forms. Leonya was telling us one evening how he had taken one of our big dugout canoes with an outboard motor to the mainland. It had been a foggy day, and he was much concerned about a string of rocks that jutted out from the coast of the mainland. Much to his relief, he suddenly heard the engine slow down. He knew then that he had entered the mouth of a small river, and in no time had the boat secured on the river's bank.

Reimar and Mina complimented Leonya on his seamanship. Their confidence in his ability to cope with anything was absolute. I thought about it for a while. I felt there was something wrong with the story. Finally, I put it into words: "I don't see why the engine should have slowed down," I objected. Leonya started very patiently. "Of course it slowed down. It had to labor against the current, so it slowed down. Have you ever walked up a mountain?" He said it so calmly, so slowly, I knew he was on edge. I was forever casting doubt on what they held to be true, and this time I was challenging something that would have been obvious to a child. I was aware of my unpopular role, but I could not keep quiet. "I think the boat would have moved more slowly upstream, but the engine would have kept going at the same rate. And since you didn't see the shore, you wouldn't have known the difference."

There were a few more exchanges like this after which Leonya left in a huff. Reimar made a pronouncement, quoting as I recall, some bit of Eastern wisdom saying that he who wins an argument very likely has lost the truth. Mina found a kinder way of expressing it. "It is not always what the intellect tells us," she said. "Sometimes intuition is a better guide. I understand even Einstein has been shown to be wrong."

At any rate, Leonya and I barely talked to one another for weeks. It was not rationality versus intuition as Mina had pictured it. My argument was intuitive also, since I didn't know then about Galilean relativity, of which this incident happened to be a good example.

The initial phases of the war in Europe had little effect on life in Garapocaia. Poland was overrun before news reached the island that the war had started. Then came a period of relative inactivity when French and German armies faced each other across seemingly impenetrable lines. When I commented on the strange calm, Reimar explained that this wasn't strange at all. "The real war is a war of ideas," he said, "and it's all going on *up there.*" I knew he was referring to the hierarchy above us. Had he been getting conflicting messages lately? I asked him where the Tibetan stood, but he only smiled, regarding it evidently as a silly question.

He was, of course, tragically wrong about the war. It was not long before the battlefronts erupted. By then I had left Garapocaia for the United States, where, perhaps a year later, I received a letter from Reimar telling me that Brazil had evacuated all foreigners from the strategically located island, and that he was forced to sell the plantation. Garapocaia had been his love, almost his obsession, for over fifteen years. But now he showed little emotion at its loss. Nothing in real life ever seemed terribly important to Reimar. Life was rather a bore one had to put up with, he told me once. He then added that his horoscope told him that he would "unfortunately" have to live a long time. I am almost sure he mentioned the figure seventy-eight. And there were so many lives ahead one had to go through.

Many years later I was in Moscow for an international biophysics congress. Over a greasy sturgeon in one of the restaurants there, quite by accident I met a Brazilian. He was in the diplomatic service, and he had known Reimar and Mina. They had both died, he told me, about three or four years earlier. That would have made Reimar about seventy-eight by my reckoning.

If I did not become a mystic as a result of my experiences at Garapocaia, it was not for lack of what others would have considered "ample evidence" for the kind of things "science cannot explain." I cannot say why these events failed to convert me and, if anything, only intensified my distaste for the occult. I am left to marvel, as I did then, at how varied can be the reaction of human brains to the same world around them.

GLOSSARY

action potential—an electrical signal emitted by a neuron and sent out along its axon.

afferent—literally "carrying in"; referring to fibers that carry information toward the central nervous system. In the case of a single neuron, the fibers (dendrites) that conduct signals to the cell body.

all-or-none—the property of neurons to "fire," i.e., produce an action potential only if the signals received exceed a certain threshold. The action potentials produced are all of the same size.

alpha motoneuron—a neuron in the spinal cord whose axon triggers a skeletal muscle.

amacrine cells—a class of neurons found in the retina.

amino acids—the chemical building blocks of all protein molecules.

ascending—referring to fibers that go toward "higher" centers in the nervous system; generally the afferent, sensory pathways.

association—the bringing together of different types of sensory information, and the resulting changes in the neural network.

atomism—a philosophy which seeks to explain the behavior of complex systems in terms of simpler, repeated substructures of the system.

antonomic nervous system—a part of the nervous system that functions generally independent of conscious control (for example, control of glands, heart muscle).

axon—a single fiber along which a neuron emits its action potentials.

bilaterality—the tendency of most nervous systems to form two laterally displaced symmetric parts.

binary logic—a logical system in which variables may have one of two possible values (e.g., 0 and 1).

blindsight—a phenomenon in which visual information is received and used by the central nervous system without producing a conscious sensation.

bootstrap—in a computer the initial set of instructions that makes the computer operative. In general, a self-enhancing process or mechanism.

causality—a doctrine according to which events in nature are completely determined by those preceding them. *See also* determinism.

cell assembly—a population of interconnected neurons that forms a functional unit.

cell death—the elimination of superfluous or ectopic neurons during early stages of development.

central nervous system—the brain and spinal cord.

central sulcus—a furrow running laterally across the surface of the brain and forming the boundary between the motor cortex and the somatosensory cortex.

cerebral cortex (also neocortex or isocortex)—the outermost structure of the mammalian brain. The most recent addition in the evolution of nervous systems.

cerebral ventricles—a series of interconnected cavities in the brain, filled with cerebrospinal fluid.

chaos—the absence of order.

chaotic systems—in physics, systems whose dynamics cannot be predicted with certainty.

chiasm—a crossing of neural fiber tracts. *See* optic chiasm.

coma—the loss of consciousness.

command neuron—a neuron that exerts unique control over specific functions.

commissure—a major tract of neural fibers connecting different parts of the brain, in particular the band of 200 million fibers connecting the left and right brain hemispheres (*great* commissure) and the forward portion (*anterior* commissure).

complex cells—a class of neurons in the mammalian visual cortex.

computer simulation—a way of predicting the outcome of a process by making a computer go through analogous steps.

consciousness—a mental state involving knowledge of one's own existence and sensations.

convergence (of neural pathways)—a situation in which fibers from a larger population of neurons "converge" on a smaller structure.

corpus callosum—Latin name for the great commissure.

cortical columns—vertical structures in the cerebral cortex within which neurons are found to have very similar receptive fields.

corticofugal—referring to fibers that "descend" from the cerebral cortex, especially those returning to sensory structures.

cutaneous senses—the various senses whose receptors are located in the skin.

cybernetics—a field of study concerned with control and communication.

deoxyribonucleic acid—large chain molecule, the carrier of genetic information.

depolarization—the reduction of the potential difference across a neural membrane.

descending—referring to fibers that go toward "lower" or more peripheral centers in the nervous system; generally the efferent or motor pathways.

determinism—a doctrine according to which a given set of circumstances must always lead to the same outcome. *See also* causality.

development (also ontogeny)—the progressive changes of an organism between conception and maturity.

divergence (of neural pathways)—a situation in which fibers from a smaller population of neurons "fan out" into a larger structure.

DNA—*see* deoxyribonucleic acid.

dualism—a philosophy which distinguishes two irreducible entities, such as mind and body.

ectopic—referring to neurons or their synaptic connections which are misplaced during development.

EEG—*see* electroencephalogram.

effectors—neurons at the output end of the nervous system acting directly on muscles or glands.

efferent—literally "carrying away"; fibers that carry information away from the central nervous system. In the case of a single neuron, the axon.

electroencephalogram (EEG)—a recording of gross electrical activity of the brain obtained by electrodes attached to the outside of the skull.

encephalization—the emergence of new structures at the "head end" of the nervous system and their increasing functional role in the course of evolution.

end plate—see motor end plate.

endorphin—one of a group of neuropeptides called opioids.

engram—a physical trace of unspecified nature forming the memory of an event.

enkephalin—one of a group of neuropeptides called opioids.

enteroceptors—receptors sampling the inner "milieu" of the body.

ESP—*see* extrasensory perception.

evoked potential—electrical response of the brain to a known stimulus.

extrasensory perception (ESP)—the purported ability of an individual to receive information through means other than his senses.

feature detector—single neuron or neuron group whose activity signals the occurrence of a particular feature in the events reported by the sensors.

feature generator—single neuron or neuron group whose activity can trigger the coordinated action of several muscles.

feedback—in positive feedback the responses will amplify chance fluctuations of a variable away from a standard value. In negative feedback such fluctuations are quenched by the response.

forebrain—the most forward of three bulges from which the vertebrate brain develops.

gamma motoneuron—a neuron in the spinal cord whose axon triggers intrafusal muscles.

ganglion cells—*see* retinal ganglion cells.

genetic code—the language of nucleotide sequences in DNA that carry the genetic information.

genetic information—the information specifying the inherited characteristics of an individual.

gestalt psychology—a school of psychology.

glial cells—the most numerous of cell types in the brain. Unlike neurons, glial cells do not transmit information by electrical impulses.

glucose—a sugar used in metabolism.

gray matter—the outer portion of the cerebral cortex containing the bulk of the cell bodies.

growth cones—structures at the tips of growing neural fibers.

hemianopia—blindness over one half of the visual field.

hemifield—one half of the visual field bounded by the vertical midline.

hemisphere—the right or left brain half.

hindbrain—the most rearward of the three bulges from which the vertebrate brain develops.

hologram—an optical method of imaging in which the information is stored in a distributed manner.

holographic memory—a theory according to which memory formation is analogous to optical holograms.

homeostatic functions—controls exerted by the brain, ensuring constancy of certain variables such as body temperature, blood pressure, and others.

hormones—vital chemicals secreted internally by glands.

hypercomplex cells—a class of neurons in the mammalian visual cortex.
hyperpolarization—an increase of the normal or resting potential of a
   nerve membrane.

identity theory—*see* psychoneural identity theory.
immune response—the manufacture of antibodies by an organism invaded
   by certain chemicals or foreign cells.
indeterminacy principle—*see* uncertainty principle.
interneuron—a neuron concerned with local neural activity rather than
   transmission of signals between different parts of the nervous system.
intrafusal muscle—muscle fibers located within a muscle spindle.
isocortex—see cerebral cortex.

knee jerk—a stretch reflex.

lateral geniculate nucleus—a population of neurons in the thalamus receiving afferents from the retina and transmitting information to the
   visual cortex.
LGN—*see* lateral geniculate nucleus.
limbic system—a portion of the brain along the border of the cerebral
   cortex.
linking hypothesis—a hypothesis asserting that specific neural activities
   (brain states) can be paired or linked with specific mental states.
lobotomy—the surgical removal of one of the brain lobes, often the
   frontal lobe (frontal lobotomy).

machine—in general, a man-made device or mechanism. According to N.
   Wiener, "a device for converting incoming messages into outgoing
   messages."
macroscopic—pertaining to objects of "everyday" or large size; consisting
   of many atoms.
macrostate—a description of a macroscopic system that neglects microscopic detail.
macroworld—the world of macroscopic systems.
masking—the suppression of the perception of one stimulus by another
   stimulus.
   backward masking—the suppression of the perception of an earlier
      stimulus by a later one.
materialism—a philosophy which seeks to explain all phenomena by the
   physical interactions of material bodies.
memory—a physical trace, or engram, caused by a past event which allows us to recall that event.
microcosm—or microworld, the world of microscopic systems.

microelectrode—a small device that is able to make electrical contact with a single neuron and monitor its activity.

microscopic—very small; on the scale of atoms and molecules.

microstate—a description of a system detailing all microscopic phenomena.

microstructure—microscopic details of the structure of a system.

microworld—*see* microcosm.

mind-body problem—read the book.

ministate—a state intermediate between a macrostate and a microstate.

monism—a philosophy which attempts to explain all phenomena by a single principle.

motoneuron—an effector neuron whose axon terminates on a muscle fiber.

motor cortex—a part of the cerebral cortex which sends fibers to motoneurons in the spinal cord.

motor end plate—the synaptic terminal of a motoneuron; located on a muscle fiber.

muscle spindle—a receptor organ located within skeletal muscles to sense muscle tension.

neocortex—*see* cerebral cortex.

nerve cell—*see* neuron.

nerve fibers—another name for axons.

nerve growth factor (NGF)—a chemical produced by the body that promotes proliferation of neurons during development.

NGF—*see* nerve growth factor.

neural code—the language that expresses the recorded sensory phenomena in terms of the activity of neurons in the central nervous system.

neural fibers—*see* nerve fibers.

neural identity theory—*see* psychoneural identity theory.

neural net—a part of the nervous system viewed as a network of interconnected neurons.

neuromuscular junction—the synapse linking the axon of a motoneuron with a muscle fiber. *See also* motor end plate.

neuron (also nerve cell)—highly specialized cell consisting of dendrites, soma, and axon. Main constituent of all nervous systems.

neuropeptides—a group of molecules occurring naturally in the brain and consisting of small chains of amino acids.

neurotransmitter—a chemical that is released by one neuron and causes electrical changes in another. The exchange occurs at the synapse.

nucleic acid—a large molecule made up of nucleotides. DNA and RNA are examples.

nucleotide—one of a number of chemicals that form the building blocks of nucleic acids.

ontogeny (also development)—the progression of an individual from conception to maturity.

opiates—chemicals with a morphine-like structure and physiological effect. Many are found in opium.

opioids—morphine-like substances found in the brain.

optic chiasm—the partial crossing of the optic nerves.

optic nerve—a tract of neural fibers leading from the retina to the LGN.

panpsychism—a school of thought in which *all* material objects are endowed with mindlike properties.

peptides—*see* neuropeptides.

phantom limb—the sensation of pain seemingly originating in a previously amputated limb.

photoreceptors—specialized cells in the retina (rods and cones) which convert energy from absorbed light into electrical signals.

phylogeny—the progression of life-forms along evolutionary lines.

physical state—a description of a material system—e.g., the brain—in terms of measurable parameters.

pluralism—a philosophy which postulates the existence of two or more irreducible components.

pneuma theory—an ancient theory attributing brain function to the flow of fluids in cerebral ventricles.

positron emission tomography (PET)—an experimental technique for imaging cross sections of the active brain.

postsynaptic potential (PSP)—a change in the membrane potential of a neuron brought about by the arrival of an action potential at an afferent synapse. PSP's may be excitatory or inhibitory.

proprioceptive—sensing part of one's own body.

protein—a large biomolecule made up of a string of amino acids.

psychoneural identity theory a theory asserting that every mental state is identical with a particular physical state of the brain.

psychoneural linking hypothesis—the assumption that mental and physical states are "linked" or paired.

psychophysical identity theory—*see* psychoneural identity theory.

pyramidal tract—a tract of neural fibers descending from the motor cortex and ultimately concerned with the control of skeletal muscles.

quantum mechanics—a contemporary physical theory replacing classical mechanics.

RAS—*see* reticular activating system.

readiness potential—a signal appearing in the EEG prior to voluntary action.

receptive field—*see* visual receptive field.

receptors—specialized cells that convert stimuli (light, pressure, temperature, etc.) into electrical signals.

reductionism—a method of explaining complex phenomena by relating their more elementary components and using fundamental physical laws.

reflex—*see* reflex arc.

reflex arc—a chain of interacting neurons leading from receptors to motoneurons.

relay cells (or neurons)—neurons whose axons convey neural information to remote parts of the brain.

relay nuclei—neural structures or populations that send axon bundles to other parts of the brain.

REM sleep—a form of sleep marked by rapid eye movements; the dream stage.

resting potential—the potential or voltage across the inactive neural membrane.

reticular activating system (RAS)—a brain structure that extends from the brainstem to the thalamus. RAS damage leads to unconsciousness (coma).

retina—a multiple sheet of neurons enveloping the back of the eye and conveying visual information from photoreceptors to retinal ganglion cells.

retinal ganglion cells—a layer of neurons in the retina.

ribonucleic acids (RNA)—a class of biomolecules made up of chains of more elementary units, the ribonucleotides.

RNA—*see* ribonucleic acids.

scotoma—a blind region in the visual field.

self-organizing system—a system that adapts its structure in response to its function.

self-reference—a logical loop, often the source of contradictions or indeterminacies.

sensation—a phenomenon observed by introspection, ordinarily resulting from sensory stimulation.

sensors—specialized organs designed to convert various forms of incident energy into neural messages. *See also* receptors.

sensory cortex—a portion of the cerebral cortex that receives sensory information (e.g., visual cortex, auditory cortex, somatosensory cortex, etc.).

sensory feedback—neural signals which are triggered by sensory stimuli and, in turn, affect the processing of further stimulation.

sensory-motor brain—a simplified view of the brain as an input-output system.

simple cells—a class of neurons in the mammalian visual cortex.

simulation—*see* computer simulation.

skeletal muscle—a muscle involved in limb movement.

soma—the cell body of a neuron.

somatosensory—pertaining to body sensations (skin, joints, muscles, etc.).

speech area—a part of the cerebral cortex involved in the production or interpretation of speech.

spinal reflex—a sensory stimulus causing muscle action through neural connections in the spinal cord.

split brain—brain after surgery in which the *corpus callosum* is transsected. Surgery performed in severe cases of epilepsy.

spontaneous activity—neural activity in the absence of stimulation.

S-R approach—an attempt to understand brain functioning by studying stimulus-response characteristics.

stretch reflex—a reflex in which the stretching of a muscle fiber by external means causes it to respond with a contraction.

sulcus—a furrow on the surface of the brain. *See* central sulcus.

synapse—a junction between two neurons. In most synapses the two neural membranes are separated by a very narrow gap. Signals are transmitted in the form of chemicals. *See neurotransmitter.*

synaptic facilitation—a possible mechanism for memory storage, in which certain synapses in the neural net are strengthened.

synaptic vesicles—small spherical structures at synapses, containing the neurotransmitter molecules.

thalamus—a large mass of neurons lying below the cerebral cortex.

thermal motion—the continuous random movement of molecules, with average speeds depending on temperature.

thermal noise—small random signals caused by thermal motion.

threshold—the minimum signal or membrane depolarization which causes a neuron to emit an action potential.

transducer—a device that converts energy from a stimulus into a suitable response.

transmitter—*see* neurotransmitter.

triune brain—an expression describing what are, according to one theory, the three main components of the human brain.

turbulence—a chaotic physical phenomenon occurring in fluid flow.

U-fiber—a neural fiber in the cerebral cortex that descends into the white matter and reemerges at another part of the same hemisphere.

uncertainty principle—a theorem in quantum mechanics, first stated by

Werner Heisenberg, according to which there exist inherent limitations in the precision with which certain quantities can be determined.

ventricles—*see* cerebral ventricles.

vesicles—*see* synaptic vesicles.

vestibular system—sensory system in the inner ear concerned with balance.

visual cortex—part of the cerebral cortex receiving visual inputs.

visual pathways—the succession of neurons and their fibers engaged in transmitting visual information.

visual projection area—a population of neurons in the neocortex whose activity maps the pattern of light falling on the retina.

visual receptive field—for a single neuron in the visual pathway the distribution of light that produces the greatest response.

white matter—portions of the brain containing mostly neural fibers.

NOTES

Chapter 1

1. Warren S. McCulloch, American psychiatrist, physiologist, brain theoretician, and poet. He is best known for his work on the logical capabilities of networks of neuron-like elements. A collection of his work has appeared under the title *Embodiments of Mind*, MIT Press, Cambridge, Mass., 1965.

2. René Descartes, French scientist, mathematician, and philosopher, viewed mind and body as separate entities (dualism) with the body governed by mechanistic laws (*Tractatus de Homine*, Leyden, 1662). For a discussion of Descartes' contributions see, e.g., H. Kearney: *Science and Change, 1500–1700*. World University Library, New York, 1971.

3. Gilbert Ryle, English materialist philosopher. See, for example, Ryle's *The Concept of Mind*, Barnes & Noble, New York, N.Y., 1949.

4. The quotation is taken from J. Z. Young: *Doubt and Certainty in Science: A Biologist's Reflections on the Brain*, Oxford, 1960. Young is a contemporary British neurophysiologist.

5. Only some fragments are preserved of the writings of the so-called pre-Socratic philosophers. Most of our knowledge comes from commentaries of later philosophers, especially Aristotle. The quotation given here is one of the few fragments by Democritus (c. 460–370 B.C.) Contemporary studies: *The Presocratics*, P. Wheelwright (ed.) Bobbs-Merrill Co., Inc., Indianapolis, Ind., 1960, *The Pre-Socratics*, A.P.D. Mourelatos (ed.), Anchor Books, Garden City, N.Y., 1974.

6. The statement is by John Burnet, *Early Greek Philosophy*, A. & C. Black, London, 1930.

7. The quotation is from John Dalton's *A New System of Chemical Philosophy,* London, 1842. This classic treatise is considered the foundation of scientific atomism.

8. George Sarton, introductory essay in Joseph Needham's *Science, Religion, and Reality.* Braziller, New York, N.Y., 1955.

9. Theodore Roszak: *The Making of a Counter Culture,* Doubleday, Garden City, N.Y., 1969.

10. *Vernon Reynolds: The Biology of Human Action,* W. H. Freeman, San Francisco, Calif., 1976.

Chapter 2

1. Vesalius: Preface to *De corporis humani fabrica,* 1543.

2. The quotation is from *The Notebooks of Leonardo da Vinci,* (English edition by E. MacCurdy), Braziller, New York, N.Y., 1956, p. 166.

3. John von Neumann: *The Computer and the Brain,* Yale Univ. Press, New Haven, Conn., 1958.

4. The quotation is from Norbert Wiener's introduction to *Nerve, Brain, and Memory Models,* N. Wiener and J. P. Schadé (eds.) Elsevier, Amsterdam, 1963.

5. See Chapter 1, note 1, on McCulloch. The paper mentioned here is included in his collection *Embodiments of Mind.*

6. Valentino Braitenberg: "Thoughts on the cerebral cortex," *Journal Theoretical Biology 46:* 421, 1974.

7. O. D. Creutzfeldt: "The neocortical link: thoughts on the generality of structure and function of the neocortex," in *Architecture of the Neocortex,* M.A.B. Brazier and H. Petsche (eds.), Raven, New York, N.Y., 1978.

8. C. G. Gross, D. B. Bender, and E. C. Rocha-Miranda: "Visual receptive fields in inferotemporal cortex of the monkey," *Science 166:* 1303, 1969.

Chapter 3

1. M.B.V. Roberts: "The rapid response of Myxicola infundibulum," *Journal Marine Biol. Ass. U.K. 42:* 527, 1962.

2. H. B. Barlow: "Single units and sensation: a neuron doctrine for perceptual psychology?" *Perception 1:* 371, 1972.

3. Steven Rose: *The Conscious Brain,* Knopf, New York, N.Y., 1974.

4. George Somjen: *Sensory Coding in the Mammalian Nervous System,* Appleton-Century-Crofts, New York, N.Y., 1972.

5. N. A. Lassen, D. H. Ingvar, and E. Skinhøj: "Brain function and blood flow," *Scientific American 239:* 62, 1978.

6. S. C. Palay: "Principles of cellular organization in the nervous system," in *The Neurosciences,* Quarton, Melnechuk, and Schmitt, (eds.), Rockefeller Press, New York, N.Y., 1967.

7. Jacques Monod: *Chance and Necessity,* Knopf, New York, N.Y., 1971. Monod, molecular biologist and Nobel laureate, has expressed his scientific philosophy in this very lucidly written book.

8. K. S. Lashley: "In search of the engram," *Symp. Soc. Exp. Biol. 4:* 454, 1950.

9. The holographic theory of memory is expounded in a book entitled *Shufflebrain,* by Paul Pietsch, Houghton Mifflin, Boston, Mass., 1980.

10. W. Ritchie Russell: *Brain, Memory, Learning,* Clarendon Press, Oxford, 1959.

11. Donald O. Hebb: *The Organization of Behavior,* Wiley, New York, N.Y., 1949.

12. E. Harth and S. Edgar: "Association by synaptic facilitation in highly damped neural nets," *Biophys. Journal 7:* 689, 1967.

Chapter 4

1. See Chapter 1, note 1.

2. William James: *Principles of Psychology,* Henry Holt, New York, N.Y., 1980.

3. Niels Bohr has frequently addressed the question of what implications modern physics has for other fields of knowledge, particularly for the life sciences. The point made here is from his essay "Light and Life," which appeared in his collection *Atomic Physics and Human Knowledge,* Wiley, New York, N.Y., 1958. This volume also contains the article "Biology and Atomic Physics" referred to in Chapter 6.

4. See Chapter 2, note 2.

5. Michael S. Gazzaniga and J. E. LeDoux, *The Integrated Mind,* Plenum, New York, N.Y., 1978.

6. S. J. Diamond and D. A. Blizard (eds.): *Evolution and Lateralization of the Brain,* N. Y. Acad. of Sciences, New York, N.Y., 1977.

7. W. Maxwell Cowan: "The development of the brain," *Scientific American 241:* 112, 1979.

8. W. Maxwell Cowan: "Selection and control in neurogenesis," in *The Neurosciences, Fourth Study Program,* F. O. Schmitt and F. G. Worden (eds.), MIT Press, Cambridge, Mass., 1979.

9. A series of studies on the effect of external, i.e., nongenetic, factors on brain structure was published in *The Neurosciences, Fourth Study Program,* a collection of articles reporting recent findings from various fields of brain research, edited by F. O. Schmitt and F. G. Worden, MIT Press, 1979. The articles on "epigenetic" effects are by P. H. Patterson ("Epigenetic influences in neuronal development"), J. Diamond ("The regulation of nerve sprouting by extrinsic influences"), G. Lynch and R. M. Akers ("Extrinsic influences on the development of efferent topographies in mammalian brain"), and R. A. Gorski ("Long term hormonal modulation of neuronal structure and function").

10. Marcus Jacobson: *The Formation of Nervous Connections,* Academic Press, New York, N.Y., 1970.

11. E. R. Macagno, V. Lopresti, and C. Levinthal: "Structure and development of neuronal connections in isogenic organisms," *Proc. Nat. Acad. of Sci. 70:* 57, 1973.

12. Paul McLean: "On the evolution of three mentalities," in *New Dimensions in Psychiatry: A World View,* Vol. II, S. Arieti and G. Chrzanokowski (eds.), Wiley, New York, N.Y., 1977.

13. David Hubel and Torsten Wiesel have been carrying out the most extensive studies of the mammalian visual cortex. A review of their findings by D. Hubel and T. Wiesel entitled "Brain Mechanisms of Vision" appeared in *Scientific American 241:* 150, 1979.

14. L. Weiskrantz, E. K. Warrington, D. M. Sanders, and J. Marshall: "Visual capacity in the hemianopic field following restricted occipital ablation," *Brain 97:* 709, 1974.

15. T. Torjussen: "Visual processing in cortically blind hemifields," *Neuropsychologia 16:* 15, 1978.

16. Ragnar Granit: *The Purposive Brain,* MIT Press, Cambridge, Mass., 1977.

17. J. K. Stevens: "The corollary discharge: is it a sense of position or a sense of space?" *The Behav. and Brain Sciences 1:* 163, 1978.

18. W.J.H. Nauta: "Anatomical Organization of Pain Pathways in the Central Nervous System," in *Opiate Receptor Mechanisms,* S. H. Snyder and S. Matthysse (eds.), *Neurosciences Research Program Bulletin 13:*84, 1975.

19. H. Akil, D. J. Mayer, and J. C. Liebeskind: "Antagonism of stimulation-produced analgesia by naloxone, a narcotic antagonist," *Science 191:* 961, 1976.

20. J. Hughes: "Isolation of an endogenous compound from the brain with pharmacological properties similar to morphine," *Brain Research 88:* 295, 1975.

Chapter 5

1. P. Tynan and R. Sekuler: "Moving visual phantoms: a new contour completion effect," *Science 188:* 951, 1975.

2. R. M. Warren: "Perceptual restoration of missing speech sounds," *Science 167:* 392, 1970.

3. Kurt Koffka: *Principles of Gestalt Psychology,* Harcourt, New York, N.Y., 1935.

4. James J. Gibson: "The theory of affordances," in *Perceiving, Acting and Knowing,* R. Shaw and J. Bransford (eds.), Wiley, New York, N.Y., 1977.

5. E. Gibson and R. D. Walk: "The visual cliff," *Scientific American 202:* 64, 1960.

6. L. Festinger: *A Theory of Cognitive Dissonance,* Stanford Univ. Press, Stanford, Calif., 1957.

7. L. Deecke, B. Grötzinger, and H. H. Kornhuber: "Voluntary finger movement in man, cerebral potentials and theory," *Biolog. Cybernetics 23:* 99, 1976.

8. W. Singer: "Control of thalamic transmission by corticofugal and ascending reticular pathways in the visual system," *Physiological Review 57:* 386, 1977.

9. Karl Pribram: "How is it that sensing so much we can do so little?" in *The Neurosciences, Third Study Program,* MIT Press, Cambridge, Mass., 1974.

10. E. Harth: "Visual perception: a dynamic theory," *Biolog. Cybernetics 22:* 169, 1976.

11. E. Harth and E. Tzanakou: "Alopex: a stochastic method for determining visual receptive fields," *Vision Res. 14:* 1475, 1974.

12. T. W. Pietsch and D. B. Grobecker: "The compleat angler: aggressive mimicry in an Antennariid anglerfish," *Science 201:* 369, 1978.

13. Note 10.

14. The discussion on pages 178–180 on a modern version of the dualist philosophy of mind and body refers to a book entitled *The Self and Its Brain* by K. R. Popper and J. C. Eccles (Springer International, Berlin, 1977). Sir John Eccles is a neurophysiologist and Nobel laureate. Karl Popper is a well-known contemporary philosopher of science.

15. Note 7.

16. B. F. Skinner: *Beyond Freedom and Dignity,* Knopf, New York, N.Y., 1971.

17. Jason Brown: *Mind, Brain, and Consciousness,* Academic Press,

New York, N.Y., 1977. In connection with our discussion on pages 185–186, see especially pages 83–85 and 94–97.

18. Sir Charles Sherrington (1861–1952) was one of the most influential early neurophysiologists. His two most frequently quoted works are *Integrative Action of the Nervous System*, Yale Univ. Press, New Haven, Conn., 1906, and *Man on His Nature,* Cambridge Univ. Press, New York, N.Y., 1951.

19. R. Efron: "The Effect of Handedness on the Perception of Simultaneity and Temporal Order," *Brain 86:* 261, 1963.

20. This point is discussed by Michael S. Gassaniga and J. E. LeDoux in *The Integrated Mind.* (See Chapter 4, note 5.)

21. Michael S. Gazzaniga: *The Bisected Brain*, Appleton-Century-Crofts, New York, N.Y., 1970.

22. Note 20.

23. Benjamin Libet: "Subjective referral of the timing for a conscious sensory experience," *Brain 102:* 193, 1979.

24. Erwin Schrödinger: *What Is Life?* and *Mind and Matter,* Cambridge Univ. Press, New York, N.Y., 1944.

Chapter 6

1. See Chapter 5, (note 23).

2. Robert Shaw: "Strange attractors, chaotic behavior and information flow," *Zeitschrift f. Naturforschung* A36: 80, 1981.

3. Douglas Hofstadter: *Gödel, Escher, Bach: An Eternal Golden Braid,* Basic Books, New York, N.Y., 1979.

4. B. Russell and A. N. Whitehead: *Principia Mathematica,* Cambridge University Press, 1960.

5. Vladimir Lefebvre: *The Structure of Awareness* (English translation by A. Rapoport), Sage Publications, Beverly Hills, Calif., 1977.

6. Tom Wicker: "Terror in Disguise," *The New York Times*, August 24, 1980.

7. Note 5.

8. J. A. Wheeler and C. M. Patton: "Is physics legislated by cosmogony?" in *The Encyclopedia of Ignorance,* R. Duncan and M. Weston-Smith (eds.), Pergamon, New York, N.Y., 1977.

9. F. J. Dyson: "Time without end: physics and biology in an open universe," *Reviews of Modern Physics 51:* 447, 1979.

10. Eugene P. Wigner: "The place of consciousness in modern physics," in *Consciousness and Reality*, C. Musès and A. M. Young (eds.), Avon, New York, N.Y., 1974.

11. The story of Schrödinger's cat goes back to an article in the Ger-

man scientific periodical *Naturwissenschaften.* For a more recent account, see B. S. DeWitt, *Physics Today,* September, 1970.

12. B. d'Espagnat: "The quantum theory and reality," *Scientific American 241:* 158, 1979.

13. See Chapter 4, note 3.

Chapter 7

1. The anecdote about Trembley and his influence on French materialism is based on an article by A. Vartanian: "Trembley's polyp, LaMettrie, and 18th century French materialism," in *Roots of Scientific Thought,* P. P. Wiener and A. Noland (eds.), Basic Books, New York, N.Y., 1957.

2. Ludwig Boltzmann: *Theoretical Physics and Philosophical Problems,* D. Reidel Publishers, Boston, Mass., 1974.

3. Norbert Wiener: *God and Golem, Inc.,* MIT Press, Cambridge, Mass., 1964.

4. See Chapter 6, note 9.

5. See Chapter 6, note 5.

6. Henrik Ibsen: *Peer Gynt* (English translation by M. Meyer), Anchor Books, Garden City, N.Y., 1963.

7. Pico della Mirandola: *Oration on the Dignity of Man* (English translation by A. R. Caponigri), Gateway Eds., Inc., Chicago, Ill. 1956.

8. D. O. Hebb: "A problem of localization," *The Behav. and Brain Sciences 3:* 357, 1978.

9. Herbert Feigl: "The Mental and the Physical," Univ. of Minnesota Press, Minneapolis, 1967.

10. The quotations by Owen St. John, as well as Leibnitz's comment on Hume are taken from St. John's article, "Nature, Life and Mind," in a collection of essays entitled *Beyond Chance and Necessity,* J. Lewis (ed.), Humanities Press, Atlantic Highlands, N.J., 1974.

11. Among the many surprises of modern physics is the finding that vacuum can no longer be regarded as the absence of everything. For a semitechnical discussion of this problem see Chapter 6, note 8.

INDEX

particle-wave duality, 69, 222
pattern completion, 156
Penfield, Wilder, 99, 197
peptides, *see* neuropeptides
perception, 34, 70–73, 99–100,
    133, 155–165, 184, 236
    as direct process, 160–163
    interpretation of reality and,
    156–160
    seeing vs., 155
perceptron, 58
peripheral neurons, 98
permanence, 15, 20, 22, 30–31,
    117
PET, *see* positron emission to-
    mography
"Petrov and Sidorov," 217–219
phantom limb, 149
photoreceptors, 49, 119, 120,
    121, 124, 125, 131, 146,
    156
phylogeny, 103–106
physicalists, 26–27
physical state, 238, 239
Piaget, Jean (1896–1980),
    Swiss psychologist, 117,
    170
Pico della Mirandola, Count
    Giovanni (1463–1494),
    Italian writer, 233–234
Pietsch, T. W., 176
pineal body, 42, 237
Pitts, Walter, 57
pituitary gland, 46, 152, 153
Planaria, see flatworms
Planck, Max (1858–1947),
    German physicist, 24
pleasure, 182
pluralism, 22, 184
pneuma theory, 38, 153
"pontifical neuron," 68
Popper, Karl, 240

positron emission tomography
    (PET), 77
postsynaptic potential, 51, 52,
    53–54, 59, 212
prefrontal cortex, 75
pre-Socratic philosophers, 22, 23
Pribram, Karl, 173, 174
Principia Mathematica (Russell
    and Whitehead), 215
Principles of Psychology
    (James), 100
prisoner's problem, 216–217
problem solving, 197
programs, 55, 56, 232
projection, 28, 99–100, 145, 169
promissory materialism, 240
proprioceptive schema, 168,
    169, 171, 174, 185
proprioceptive system, 137
protein, 78, 94, 96–97, 114,
    151, 152, 207
psychokinesis, internal, 178
psychological self, physical self
    vs., 17–18
psychoneural identity theory,
    see psychophysical identity
    theory
psychoneural linking hypothesis,
    239
psychophysical identity theory,
    29, 34, 72, 83, 227, 237–
    240
Puccetti, Roland, 192, 193
pulse logic, 70, 73
pyramidal tract, 47, 140–141,
    143, 167, 171

quantum mechanics, 24, 31, 184,
    204, 208, 219, 221–226,
    240
quarks, 33, 194, 204